KE

Moving

KEEP

Young

Gentle
Yoga Exercises

MARGARET
GRAHAM

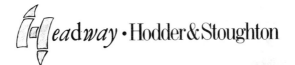

Headway · Hodder & Stoughton

British Library Cataloguing in Publication Data

Graham, Margaret
  Keep Moving, Keep Young: Gentle Yoga
  Exercises for Older People. – 2Rev.ed
  I. Title
  613. 70460846

ISBN 0 340 621176

First published in Great Britain by Unwin® Paperbacks, an imprint of Unwin Hyman
Limited in 1988
Updated and published by Hodder Headline, 1995

Impression number   10 9 8 7 6 5 4 3 2 1
Year   1999 1998 1997 1996 1995

Typeset by Wearset, Boldon, Tyne and Wear.
Printed in Great Britain for Hodder & Stoughton Educational, a division of Hodder
Headline Plc, 338 Euston Road, London NW1 3BH by Page Bros (Norwich) Ltd.

CONTENTS

This book is dedicated to past and present residents of Ifield Park Home for the Elderly and older students in Crawley, Roffey and Horsham. They have been such willing guinea pigs and inspired so many of us by their hard work and enthusiasm.

FOREWORD

Keep Moving, Keep Young is a lovely book, designed with the older generation in mind, and full of sensible, practical advice, written in no-nonsense language. As we approach the end of the twentieth century, more and more people are seeing the wisdom of taking responsibility for their own state of health. Ageing is no longer seen as a disease, just another stage of life to be valued and understood. Any book which helps to improve the quality of our lives as we grow older, but which does not set out to replace the support of a medical team where it is necessary, has got to be good news, and this is just what *Keep Moving, Keep Young* is intended to do.

Looking back, I remember when Margaret first approached The British Wheel of Yoga some eleven years ago with an idea for a booklet aimed at the older and less-able student – we had little idea that *It's Never Too Late* would become one of our most popular booklets. The follow-up was its big sister, *Keep Moving, Keep Young*, now updated in its second edition. I am delighted that a new generation of golden oldies will have the opportunity of discovering yoga, and have no doubt they will find this book just as inspiring as the first readers did. I wish them all a long and happy journey through the wisdom years.

Diana Kendall

Former chairman of the British Wheel of Yoga and currently
Secretary General to The European Yoga Union

September 1994

PREFACE

This book sets out to show that older people can benefit and enjoy gentle exercise and relaxation whatever their age or limitations.

The basis is yoga, but there are no headstands or lotus positions here, nor is there any mystique involved. The slow, smooth movements, the use of breathing and relaxation, make it ideal for the older population – even if they haven't exercised since 'physical jerks' in the school playground.

The medical profession is anxious for people of all ages to become active, to keep moving. Facilities abound – swimming pools, athletic clubs, keep fit, aerobic and yoga groups. Most are for the young to middle-aged population. A few are for the 'not so young' or 'over 60s'. But what about the over 70s? The over 80s? Even the over 90s? For this important and growing proportion of people there seems little provision. And yet for them keeping moving is probably most vital of all. And what if you're housebound or don't relish activities *en masse?* What if you don't possess a tracksuit (men), leotard or even a pair of slacks (ladies)? Supposing you've enjoyed years of sport or keep fit and are finding it harder to get there or keep up?

Older people don't want to be left out of the fitness boom. They may want to keep fit but are scared or don't know how. Many will not be willing, or even able, to get down on the floor.

Here is a guide, tested and evolved by people of 70 to 100 years. The basic exercises are performed seated, others standing with a chair for support. There's no special equipment or clothing needed. There are suggestions to help you relax, as well as mental exercises such as concentration and visualisation which are fun to try, can have real physical benefits and help keep the grey matter ticking over. The approach is positive, the accent on what you *can* do.

This book can be used in different ways by different readers. You may be 'getting on' and looking for something you can do quietly at home which will help you to keep moving, loosen up, relax, etc. You may be hoping to find something your local club or group of friends can do together. Perhaps you have an elderly friend or relative you would like to help, without being too pushy. Or you may already be working with this age-group in a club or home and are looking for helpful ideas. Or you teach a keep fit, yoga or similar group and need to find suggestions for your older members or students who have temporary or permanent limitations. Whatever the reason, this book should be a useful aid, along with your own sensitivity and common sense.

The method of using the book will vary. You may like to read it straight through and get the general idea before trying specific exercises or routines – this really is the best way. However, many of us are more impatient or short of time and prefer to 'dip in', to find something for a particular problem (my aching back, Dad's arthritic hands). You will find that the exercises are listed from head to toe in Chapters 6 to 11 to help you find them. However, if you do intend to dip in, please make sure you read Chapter 5 first which gives very important practical advice.

In Appendix 1 you will find a variety of programmes, from a basic programme to a number of programmes in which a range of individual exercises have been put together to make varied and balanced half-hour sessions.

And if you are still left with questions, why not turn to Appendix 2, Questions People Ask. Other people will undoubtedly have had the same queries as you, and we have tried to answer some of the most common questions here.

Your doctor should be able to advise you about exercising, taking into account your own individual state of health, but make sure you explain the gentle nature of our exercise – take the book along if necessary. Otherwise he or she may be under the impression that you're going to attempt a marathon, tie yourself in knots or do the splits! Just as conventional yoga students are advised to seek their doctor's approval before starting lessons, so it is important that older students too should put their doctor in the picture.

There's no need to consult the doctor though before trying the little test in Chapter 3. It's all about tuning in and discovering things about yourself that may have gone unnoticed for as long as half or even three-quarters of a century. Try it. What you discover will be of great benefit in your future gentle exercise programme and, more importantly, in your daily life.

ACKNOWLEDGEMENTS

I am indebted to the British Wheel of Yoga – its members, teachers and teacher trainers. Without them this project and book could never have existed. I would like to give love and thanks to all those teachers with whom I have studied. They have shared their knowledge, experience and enthusiasm so generously, allowing me in turn to pass on and adapt their teachings to the needs of older people.

Firstly then my thanks to Gill Lloyd, who laid the foundation of good yoga practice and gave shape to the original idea of a basic programme. Gill's classes continue to be a source of recreation and stimulation. And to my tutors and friends Greta and Ken Bennett. And to Joy Burling and Jean Oddy, in appreciation of their special skills in teaching therapeutic yoga, making valuable contributions to such items as 'breathing', chest complaints, back pain and also to visualisation. To Dr Barbara Brosnan and her 'floor squad' of handicapped people who demonstrated the wonderful power of yoga linked to dedication and hard work. To Philip Jones, for his good advice on breathing when I started teaching and for his contribution to the chapter 'Breath of Life'. To Ken Thompson and Don Stevens for their advice and encouragement, Dottie Hook for her special care and to Lindy Gillam, Di Kendall and all those involved in the production of *It's Never too Late*, published by the British Wheel of Yoga. And to cover models Jane Monger, Gladis 'Robbie' Robinson and John Johnston.

I appreciate the practical help and advice given by practitioners of complementary medicine, including Matthew Manning, Arvid Willen, Brenda Mills and Sue Czornenkyj, as well as assistance given by Dr Ivan Clout who encouraged the original 'experiment' at Ifield Park and kindly cast a professional eye over the manuscript. Also to Professor Michael Hall, Dr Joan Bassey, Dr Dorothy Jerome, Dr Marilyn Glenville, Dr Angela Gurner, H Soni, Margie Polden, Thais de Lima Resende, Gill Avery and Judith Williams, all of whom added their expertise. A big thank-you to Doreen Montgomery for her help and encouragement, to Rowena Gaunt and Sue Hart.

I owe much to my father, Harold Goodwin, founder of Ifield Park, a pioneer in his field, giving elderly people the independence, care and self-respect which should be the right of every individual, regardless of age. And to Mother and my sister Frances who are continuing his work.

My thanks to my husband David, and my children Fiona, Jenny and Alasdair. Their support and sense of humour (not to mention some original spelling) made it all an adventure.

The biggest thanks of all goes to our greatest teachers – the students, to whom this book is dedicated.

Formal acknowledgements are made to the following authors and their publishers for quotations and influence of their work:

Professor Michael Hall, W J MacLennan, M D W Lye, *The Medical Care of the Elderly*, John Wiley & Sons, Chichester;

Dr Barbara Brosnan, *Yoga for Handicapped People*, Souvenir Press, London;

Kevin Morgan & Ken Gledhill, *Managing Sleep & Insomnia in the Older Person*, Winslow Press;

Jane Madders, *Stress and Relaxation*, Positive Health Guide.

The extract from *Leisure*, by W H Davies, appears by kind permission of the Executors of the W H Davies estate.

CHAPTER 1

Use it –
don't lose it

Does someone over 60 or 70 really have to be bothered with exercise? 'Haven't I earned a rest' you may wonder, 'after years of hard work, most of it for other people?' Whatever happened to the picture of dear old white-haired granny, gently dozing in her rocking chair by the fire? Simply this: What you don't use, you lose!

If granny spent most of her day in such idyllic repose it wouldn't be long before she just wouldn't have the strength to heave herself out of her chair, let alone bring the coal in and stoke up the fire. If you have ever broken a limb and spent weeks with it encased in plaster, I'm sure you'll have noticed how the muscle shrank and how weak and useless it felt.

Think, too, how feeble you feel after a week in bed with flu. This isn't just the effects of the bug, but muscular weakness too. Inactivity will also slow down your circulation – your feet can feel really cold after an evening of sitting still, even in a cosy room. Here granny has the right idea with the rocking chair; the gentle rhythmic foot movements help to keep the circulation going in her feet and legs.

You have probably noticed that over the years hospital stays have become shorter and that after even a major operation you're got up much more quickly. It's not so much that they want to be rid of you as to keep everything in the body moving, ticking over, helping to avoid medical complications which can be aggravated by inactivity. It also lessens that feeling of general weakness, and we feel better for soon being up and about again, however much we may grumble about it at the time!

Sometimes a person suffering from a disabling condition puts **all** symptoms of stiffness and weakness down to the disease, when lack of use can be a big factor. I have seen such students improve – both physically and psychologically – by using a regular, gentle exercise routine.

KEEP MOVING

The medical profession is keen to keep older people moving. Michael Hall, professor of geriatric medicine, says that 'There is much evidence from laboratory-based studies that the elderly can improve physically and benefit from exercise just as much as the young.' He thinks that many people are brainwashed into believing that they will deteriorate simply because they are getting older – and so they do.

I'm sure you know people who don't accept that age alone is a reason for stopping a favourite activity, or starting a new one. Well before the jogging craze I remember a man of 90 who ran round the block every day, heedless of the weather, shorts flapping, white beard trailing in the early morning breeze. Neighbours tut-tutted and said it would be the death of him. They were alarmed, though, when suddenly he ceased to be seen pounding his familiar beat. Had their fears been realised? No, always restless, he'd upped and emigrated to Australia.

Such people may be the exception, but we seem to hear of more and more of them. The other year the oldest competitor to complete the London Marathon was aged 79. And it's not just running. In Los Angeles, at their Senior Olympics, competitors of 60 years and over take part in such events as high-jumping and wrestling. Nearer home, just look around your town at the age of some of the cyclists, from people fetching goods on their shoppers to some of the veterans in the local cycle club.

However, though such people prove that old age itself is not a disease, there are many who find that such vigorous activity, even if they wished to take part in it, just is not possible because of chronic disease such as arthritis, bronchitis or heart disease. So what can *they* do? There may be a tricky hip to contend with, or just climbing stairs may leave you breathless. You may be afraid to exercise in case you harm yourself or aggravate an existing medical condition. There may be a feeling that you are generally stiffening up. 'It's all right for those cocky octogenarian athletes, but *we* are simply not as young as we were. What's more we don't fancy all that energetic leaping around that keep fit exercises seem to involve. And anyway, isn't it just too late?'

IT'S NEVER TOO LATE

It's never too late, even for the frail elderly person, even for someone confined to a wheelchair. No one is too far gone to embark on the gentle exercise system based on yoga and described in this book. It is being used by many elderly people, some in their 90s. Over the past few years they have proved to themselves as well as others that they can not only attempt such exercise but really enjoy it and benefit from it. All the movements and relaxation described in this book can be done seated in a chair. If you want to try some standing postures these are described too, with a chair to hold on to if you feel a bit wobbly. There is a section on floor postures, but don't be put off if you don't want to get down there – some can be done quite effectively on, or even in, your bed. However limited your range of movement – perhaps you can only wriggle your fingers – there is always something you can work on. It is said that if you can breathe you can practise yoga.

Some other readers may be getting on in years but are still fit and leading a full and active life. Is there any point in doing these exercises? I think so. Yoga is like that lager advert – it reaches parts that others don't. It can keep those parts in good working order and also help keep you alert and topped up with energy.

WHAT IS YOGA?

But why yoga? Doesn't that mean standing on your head or sitting for hours on the floor with your legs tied in knots? 'What me, in my condition?', I can hear you saying, 'You must be joking!' And going by some publications and television programmes, you might think that the only people who can practise yoga are 20-year-old females who are double-jointed, weigh 7 stone and have a vast wardrobe of skin-tight slippery-looking costumes which leave you wondering, as one old lady put it, 'where on earth they keep their handkerchief'.

Such representations can do a disservice to yoga. True yoga can be practised by anyone. You don't have to be able to do headstands or sit in the lotus position. The basic movements and breathing patterns, deceptively simple but so important for improving health, can be practised in a chair. The only requirement is a willingness to have a go.

And why the ancient practice of yoga when there is a veritable confusion of modern exercise routines? Yoga works so well because its slow, smooth movements can be adapted to every individual. If your arm will only lift to shoulder height that's OK – you work at that level. There is plenty of time to find the fine line between effort and strain without having to worry about any sense of competition or feeling that you have to keep up with everybody else. And yoga is more than physical exercise. Our method still includes attention to posture and breathing, but mental exercise comes into it too – concentration and visualisation – and of course relaxation. In short, yoga is a complete, balanced and, above all, gentle system.

Yoga originated in India at least 2,500 years ago, and came to the West via returning soldiers and civil servants. The West has been using it for a century or so and in the last few years yoga has been used increasingly as a therapy.

THE BENEFITS OF YOGA

Ancient yogis knew many things that scientific research is now discovering for itself. For example, 'movement is life'. Doctors now recognise this and encourage people recovering from heart attacks to engage in a gradual, safe exercise programme – after all, the heart, like other muscles, needs to be kept exercised in order to function. Regular appropriate exercise on the lines of yoga has even been found to help build up bones that have become weaker (de-mineralised). This tendency – called osteoporosis – seems to affect many women after the change of life (menopause). A recent article in a medical journal recommended that for protection against osteoporosis you should have dietary supplements, sunshine, good posture, back care precautions, exercise and no smoking. It is only recently that sensitive scientific equipment has been developed which can measure such gradual changes. This verifies what many of us have always known – that movement, sports and hobbies are good for us as well as fun. What else will they discover in the future?

To keep moving is particularly important (though perhaps hardest of all) for arthritis sufferers. Working the muscles which surround an affected joint keeps them in good condition, helps protect and support the joint and improves the circulation. Of course, care must be used and a joint should never be worked while it is inflamed – that is, when it is swollen and perhaps red and hot, as well as extremely painful. Some of our most encouraging results have come from elderly students with arthritis. If you are a sufferer there is more detailed information on working with this condition (and others) in Chapter 5.

Modern medicine has also found that relaxation does you good. Relaxation in this sense means being able to sit or lie still, being able to switch off, to let go both in body and mind. Even if it is only for a few minutes, such relaxation can be as beneficial and refreshing as hours of (perhaps restless) sleep. Hospitals teach relaxation techniques to help with the treatment of all sorts of conditions, from pregnancy to anxiety states, from insomnia to asthma.

THE BASIC TECHNIQUES

So, apart from exercise and relaxation, what else will you be letting yourself in for? The answer is work on posture, breathing, concentration and visualisation – and don't be put off by the sound of these last two, you've probably been practising them for years without realising it. Sometimes I think my work is very much a case of 'teaching Granny to suck eggs'. A few words about each of these subjects, however.

Posture
As you may already know, poor posture – rounded shoulders, for example, or sitting with the back curved or not supported in the right way – can cause all sorts of aches, strains and pains, as well as aggravating existing conditions. Good posture, on the other hand, not only makes you feel better in yourself but also puts less strain on muscles and joints, and on your insides too, since nothing can function well if it is cramped up. This especially concerns the lungs, which brings us to . . .

Breathing

Learning to make good use of your breathing equipment has many benefits. It can be helpful for people who suffer from chest complaints – asthma, bronchitis or general 'chestiness' for example. Physiotherapists often treat such patients with breathing exercises. Good breathing not only helps the whole body function better, but the mind and emotions can benefit too. The chapter on breathing includes different ways of using the breath to give you more energy, to calm you down, and even to let off steam.

Concentration

As with other skills, the ability to concentrate gets better with practice. Even if you think you have a hopeless 'butterfly' mind, you'll be surprised how it can improve without you even realising it. Simply going through each exercise or posture will mean that you are having to apply yourself. For a start, you will have to think which is your left and which your right (many of us get it wrong even after years of practice – and I don't just mean the students!).

It is generally assumed that it is harder to learn as you grow older, the 'scientific' theory being that this is due to progressive loss of brain cells. 'Not true', says Dr Dorothy Jerome, who has a particular interest in this field. The loss of brain cells is only about 2½ per cent in a lifetime, and she states that 'People who exercise their faculties, who consolidate or advance their existing interests and seek new ones not only halt the decline in capacity but actually improve their performance.' My own observations certainly bear this out. Unfortunately, too many people think that you become less intelligent as you age, and this is often used to justify common errors, lapses in memory and lack of motivation. Dr Jerome believes 'All of these are experienced by any adult; middle-aged and older people use *age* to account for them.' So you *can* teach an old dog new tricks.

Practising breathing, relaxation and visualisation all provide mental exercise and help improve concentration. When I find mine lapsing (having always been a bit of a dreamer) I wonder how much worse I'd be without yoga! But why should we make such efforts to improve our concentration? If our mind is on what we are doing it helps every activity undertaken, from singing hymns to writing out the shopping list. And concentration can be a life-saver when trying to cross today's busy roads.

Visualisation

This is simply a trendy word for using your imagination, for seeing with the mind's eye. This is when being a dreamer comes in handy. Visualisation can have beneficial physical effects and is enjoyable in itself. Picturing a pleasant scene while relaxing really helps the body and mind let go, and when you come round again you're more likely to feel refreshed and happy. A lovely example of this is a student of 90 (an alert and practical woman) who looked positively radiant after a short relaxation to dreamy waltz music. 'I was dancing with such a nice young man', she explained. The glow lasted all day.

Visualisation can be helpful in postures too. Picturing a stiff limb moving freely or going into a difficult position is much more helpful than trying to force the poor thing where it doesn't want to go.

It appears that appropriate visualisation during relaxation can help people suffering from all sorts of problems, from arthritis to colitis, lack of confidence to headaches. It is a technique taught by many therapists. In this country the Bristol Cancer Help Centre is probably best known for making such excellent use of this gentle therapy.

ENJOYMENT

So now you have all sorts of reasons for having a go at this gentle exercise system. However, nothing will keep you at it if it isn't enjoyable. For a start, there is no need to tackle things in too grim and determined a manner. Though little and often is the best motto, don't be too hard on yourself if you have an off day or forget to do your exercises for a while. You can pick up again when and where you like. There's no hurry and no one to please but yourself.

And if you find yourself agreeing with all the theory behind this exercise lark but there's still a little voice at the back of your head saying 'It's all right for her to be so keen. Wait till she's my age', well, I don't blame you. So let's move on to the next chapter and see how the first elderly (but very willing) guinea pigs got on.

CHAPTER 2

THE EXPERIMENT

If you wandered into Ifield Park Home for the Elderly on a Tuesday or Thursday morning you'd probably wonder what on earth was going on. Dining chairs in a circle, 15 or more residents sitting silently, stockinged feet resting comfortably on cushions, hands in laps, eyes closed. A prayer meeting? A séance? If you thought that, you'd be rather startled by what follows. A voice rings out, 'Raise your eyebrows, screw up your eyes . . . relax. Purse your lips, give a big smile.' And you'd find yourself smiling too; you wouldn't be able to help it. We all laugh here, and another yoga class is underway.

All over the country conventional yoga classes for the 'not so young' are thriving. Postures may have to be adapted and more time allowed for the business of getting up and down from the floor, but the result is many older students who are excellent adverts for the benefits of yoga.

But introducing yoga to people in their 70s, 80s and 90s – surely that's quite a different matter? How can they effectively work the whole body (or the parts that still function) from a chair – or a wheelchair even? Can they really do relaxation like that? Might they not fall off the chair if they do? These were all questions we asked ourselves when contemplating some sort of gentle exercise and relaxation class, based on yoga, for the residents of Ifield Park.

THE BACKGROUND

In 1954 my parents, Harold and Millicent Goodwin, founded Ifield Park, a voluntary charitable home in Crawley, West Sussex. I had virtually grown up in the home and worked there for many years.

The benefits of yoga I discovered for myself as the result of a rather unorthodox prescription by my GP. He suggested it might help alleviate the backache I was suffering. It was almost with surprise that I found my back growing stronger and more supple as I attended first one, then two yoga classes a week at our local leisure centre. And there were other benefits. I found that I could start to control and relieve the migraine headaches that had plagued me since childhood. Like many students, I found the breathing exercises a bit of a bore to start with. Then I started to recognise them as a very useful tool in lessening the tension which so often underlies backache, migraine and a whole host of other 'dis-eases'.

Feeling so much better for this new lease of life and energy, I wondered if there wasn't some way of bringing similar benefits to my elderly friends at Ifield Park. Though they are the usual age range found in a residential home, the environment is such that privacy and independence are very much encouraged. The result is that residents keep lively, active and interested in day-to-day goings on – as one visitor put it, 'They've got a twinkle in their eye.' What better group to try out a new idea with? Even if the average age is 85 and they are suffering the usual infirmities associated with their years, they are a lively valuable cross-section of the community and worth a bit of effort.

So I consulted Gill Lloyd, my excellent yoga teacher. Equally enthusiastic, we put our heads together and the result was the basic programme of exercises found at the beginning of Appendix 1. All the postures and movements could be performed seated or standing with a chair for support, and could be adapted to the individual need of an elderly student. The home's doctor, Ivan Clout, encouraged the scheme, happy for his patients to be kept moving.

Then I started to get cold feet as more questions arose. Would such a class really appeal to the residents? Would the novelty wear off? Would they put enough in to get something out? Was it simply TOO LATE? Of course there was only one way to find out.

THE YOGA CLASSES

I soon felt ashamed at how completely I'd underestimated my elderly friends. Of the 70 residents, so many came to the first class it was obvious that two sessions per week would be necessary. Ifield Park is not a nursing home, so many residents are quite active; however if or when they do become more frail, they are able to stay on, so there will always be 'students' with various walking aids, and even some in wheelchairs.

Enthusiasm was high at the start and has remained unabated ever since. We soon fell into a pattern of up to 20 students at the Tuesday class, 15 on the Thursday. Some keen ones attended both, and their keenness soon paid dividends. Many residents seemed to be practising on their own, perhaps daily, in their little flatlets. They said they would twiddle fingers or toes while watching TV, do a few stretches or limbering-up movements on getting up in the morning, or go through relaxation at night instead of counting sheep.

We had been careful not to promise miracles, emphasising that any improvements would take time, but it wasn't long before the hand exercises started to show results. Lucy, over 80, found that she could now order an uncut loaf again, as she was able to grasp the knife firmly once more to slice it herself (most Ifield Park residents make their own breakfast and tea). Reg, nearly 90, took us to task for making the 'knobs' on his fingers go down so much his ring slipped off in Woolworths (quickly retrieved, thank goodness). One student thought that the eye exercises had given her a wider field of vision: 'I can see the bus appearing round the corner without turning my head.' Another said that the relaxation helped her to get to sleep without resorting to tablets so often. Several mentioned that they could reach that elusive zip at the back of the neck.

Even though improvements could have been partly psychological, it was so encouraging to hear the conversation revolving not around ailments, but improvements in health. This positive attitude was one of the more subtle changes to be observed along with the more obvious ones of better posture, balance, coordination and concentration.

Although students took their exercises seriously, there were plenty of opportunities for laughter and a sense of fun. Just try to maintain your dignity while spinning an imaginary hula-hoop round your hips, or to keep a straight face while patting your head and rubbing your tummy at the same time!

Originally I'd wondered whether visualisation techniques used during relaxation might be rather 'way out' for this age group but, once again, I was the one lacking in imagination. Picturing a favourite place, a tree, a happy scene from the past and other such suggestions all received enthusiastic comments. It does seem true that vividly picturing the past is one of the compensations of old age. Perhaps concentration is better too in those who are not leading the more hectic lives of younger people. Whatever the explanation, the attitude of these elderly students has certainly inspired many of us.

Some of our original ideas when planning these classes had to be re-thought. In the early days we found that when breathing was first introduced, simply bringing attention to the flow of their own breath caused one or two to panic and overbreathe. Taking expert advice, instead of teaching it as an isolated activity we used sequences of arm movements, emphasising the correct breathing pattern. This seemed to work well and later, when they were used to using the breath in this way, breathing exercises didn't raise such problems.

Gill and I had already decided against movement to music as this would mean that individuals could not work at their own pace. Soft background music was tried, but soon abandoned as many people (especially those with hearing aids) found it distracting. However, a variety of soothing music – such as Beethoven's Moonlight Sonata – played during the relaxation period at the end of class has been much appreciated.

Most students enjoy the social occasion of a class. Although doing exercise as a group has many advantages – 'Does your neck creak too? That's a relief, I thought I was the only one!' – it doesn't suit some so well. One lady whose movement was becoming painful and limited by arthritis stopped coming to classes because she felt so discouraged to see others progressing. Non-competitiveness is always stressed, and observed well, but this was an understandable reaction. At least she continued to practise in her own time.

The natural reticence of some older people may account for the reluctance of our class to have helpers in to lift difficult limbs, etc. It seems that they prefer the set-up of a conventional class, with a tactful hand from its teacher. This independence is something which should be respected and I think outweighs its drawbacks. Of course, if the students were all heavily handicapped, helpers would be essential.

Our classes are called 'Gentle exercise and relaxation', as I was afraid that a yoga title could put off prospective students who might associate yoga with sitting in the lotus position or standing on one's head. However, to some, especially those with family members attending conventional yoga classes, the link soon became apparent. In contrast, an enthusiastic student of 80 was heard to say 'My word, we'll be doing yoga next!' The surprise and delight on her face was a picture when she was told that she *had* been, for four months!

THE RESULTS

Word of our experiment and its success soon spread. There were articles in local papers and newsletters, and soon there was a demand for worksheets, talks and demonstrations. At various times visitors – therapists, nurses, keep fit and yoga teachers – sat in on our classes, hoping to do something similar in their own field. Friends and relatives wanted to know more, or have a go themselves. I found that I, and other yoga teachers, were being asked to set up short courses or one-off classes for over-60s clubs, church groups and adult education centres. In response to this the British Wheel of Yoga published a booklet called *It's Never Too Late*, outlining our experimental scheme and describing the exercises in detail. We were overwhelmed by the response. It was lovely to be able to tell our students of the demand for copies from all sorts of organisations, from teaching hospitals, from members of the medical profession and from complementary medical practitioners – but mostly from older people themselves. Far from being shut away from the modern world, Ifield Park and other such exercise groups were blazing the way. It's great to have an ego boost at any age and by this time of life, wise to the ways of the world, I don't think there's much harm of these celebrities getting carried away.

Following the unexpected success of this modest little book it seemed that appetites were whetted and people wanted to know more details – relaxation, breathing and all the rest. Hence the latest effort – this book.

And what of our original guinea pigs, the people in the first classes?

Some have come and gone, as is the nature of such a home. We remember with affection those who have shared our adventure. Many are still with us, some a little more frail, but undaunted. Some seem to defy time itself and, if anything, seem more active than before. Though the faces in the group may change, the spirit remains the same.

We are part of the larger yoga world, too, with visiting teachers, demonstrations by conventional classes and reciprocal visits by other elderly exercise groups.

Some of the students occasionally venture on to the floor for a course of conventional postures. For these, trousers have to be found. Lucy, nearly 90, bought her own pair, her first ever. 'I don't know', she beamed; 'Whatever would Mother have said!'

FEEDBACK

And what do the students have to say? Well, here are a few of their comments.

After half an hour's gentle exercising at our Tuesday class I can feel the blood in my veins and feel I could climb mountains. I hate to miss a class. (Audrey Robinson)

I have felt noticeable benefit from following Margaret Graham's gentle exercise routine. I am 72 and my problem is arthritis, particularly in my feet and neck and shoulder regions. I am keen to keep things moving as long as possible. The relaxation part of the routine has been most helpful in reducing the tension in the shoulders and neck, and movement there is now much more comfortable. I find that exercising in a group is not only enjoyable but a great morale-booster too. The sight of people older and more handicapped than you are, cheerfully working on their exercises, and showing very definite signs of improvement, spurs you on to even greater efforts. And when you exercise on your own the creaks in your joints can seem deafening! Do it with a group and your own creaks are only part of a chorus of everyone else's and can be disregarded.

My sister-in-law had suffered for years with arthritis in the back of her neck which was very painful and was steadily getting worse. Driving was difficult as she had to turn her shoulders to see sideways instead of just turning her head. Her doctor – out of date? – had forbidden exercises. She saw Margaret's exercise booklet and tried the head-turning exercises, and improved in just a week. Now, after a few months of daily exercise, she is able to turn her head again without having to turn her shoulders too. She is in a lot less pain and finding life a lot easier. She has changed her doctor too! Her new one thoroughly approves of her exercise routine. (Mrs Win Huss)

Over the past five years I have attended many of these 'Easy exercises for the elderly' classes and found them helpful and relaxing. During this time I have hurt myself quite badly from falls outside and my recovery has been helped by the gentle exercising and the patient care of the teacher. The 30 minutes involved is also a pleasant social interlude, plus the inevitable cup of tea.

The journey through the 80s and 90s is not an easy one and anything that promotes a wider outlook and change of thought is welcomed and *must* be beneficial. (Dorothy A Hayter)

And finally a poem by Grace Edwards that sums it all up.

Make way, make way
For the Zimmer brigade!
Some in wheelchairs,
Some without aid,
Stand back there
And let them pass!
They are on their way
To the yoga class.
They will flex their fingers
And wriggle their toes;
Stand on one leg in a tremulous pose;
Turn their heads this way
Then turn them that;
Stand against the wall
Till their backs are quite flat.
From what does all this energy derive?

It is surely the urge to stay alive,
To enjoy the simple pleasures of life
Free of anxiety, worry and strife.
Exercises over, conversation abounds;
With laughter and talk
The whole place resounds.
A successful enterprise
Good to see!
The session ends
With biscuits and tea.

UPDATE

Since this book was first published in 1988, the idea of appropriate exercise for older people has really caught on. Many have had their interest and enthusiasm captured by exercise spots on TV. It is no longer strange for, say, an 80-year-old to 'work out' from a chair. Older people are now more willing to have a go themselves. Our classes at Ifield Park and other centres have reflected this change.

Using music

A modification I have made to one of the yoga-based classes is to make more use of music. Some people respond to music in a way that far outweighs some of the difficulties that can be encountered. For the comparatively fit and active older student, it makes a change to use familiar loosening movements and stretches to lively music, or do the four-way stretch with calm, flowing music in the background. But it has been amongst the frailer students that music has really been a boon. Trying to stimulate and keep the attention of mildly confused elderly people is always a problem for those who care for them. In theory, the slow, smooth movements of yoga are ideal for even the frailest person, but if a session is too quiet and introspective, you may find that half the class has peacefully nodded off! This tendency is even worse if, unlike at Ifield Park, residents are routinely medicated into doziness.

When taking a class that's going to include some movement to music, I find it best still to run it on the same lines, starting in the yoga way with a short settling down period, then a posture check, some action breaths, stretches and loosening movements. Once the music tape is playing (Max Bygraves is a favourite), we might repeat the movements and do some other simple ones – shoulder rolling, hand clenching and stretching, heel-toe movements, clapping and often some improvisation, as the students get involved. The usual principles of not rushing or jerking and of going at your own rate apply. Some will need to move at half the rate of others, but with an alert and sensible tutor, it will be a safe and lively session. Even those who are unwilling to join in can be spotted with their toes tapping or singing along.

After this we turn off the tape and calm down again by doing a few movements that need more careful attention – head turning, tummy or pelvic floor exercises, breathing and concentration exercises. We finish with a short relaxation as usual. With an appropriate group, this method of introducing music to accompany the movements seems to work well. Both staff and relatives have commented that the residents, especially the more introverted, perk up and become more chatty after the session.

If you are interested in including some movement to music in your programme, EXTEND (their address is at the back of this book) have details and tapes. My local authority – West Sussex County Council – is far-seeing in that it runs Physical Activity to Music for the Elderly courses for carers, staff and other interested people. Let us hope that more courses on these lines will be set up in the future.

Other spin-offs

Out of our original gentle exercise classes other things have evolved too. With the cup of tea and chat after class, the conversation will sometimes turn to diet and home remedies. Older friends often comment on how these things go round in circle – many note that the household hints of their day are now recommended in the media: camomile tea to calm tummies and induce sleep, onions and garlic for colds, cod liver oil for rheumatics, and plant oils for rubbing onto stiff joints. We could produce our own *Home Herbal!*

As a result of our conversations, quite a few of the residents are making use of the old remedies again and comment on improvements noticed. After a week or two of rubbing her stiff shoulder with Olbas

oil, Mrs Holyoake lifted her arm to reach something and thought
'Ooh, that's funny, I can't usually do that!' Others have discovered
basic homoeopathic remedies and make good use of them: Arnica for
falls, Rhus Tox for rheumatic pain, Ignatia for grief, the biochemic
tissue salt Mag Phos for cramp, Bach Flower Rescue Remedy for
shock or panic. Such remedies can do no harm and I think that self-
help can so often be linked to self-esteem. Entering sheltered housing
or a residential home shouldn't mean handing yourself over body and
soul to the care of the establishment, leaving no room for
individuality or decision-making. Ifield Park is lucky in that it also
has an open-minded medical advisor.

Encouraging independence and physical fitness

Physical activity and independence in old age is something that the
Centre for Policy on Ageing advocates and encourages. This
organisation lays down guidelines for residential homes and produces
reports that provide very practical help. Since the CPA heard of our
classes, we have cooperated with them in their endeavour to list and
evaluate activities in residential homes. Modified yoga is one of the
activities the CPA would like to see available in every home. It is my
hope that eventually we shall be able to realise this ambition. Dotted
around the country there are yoga teachers working with small groups
of older people, quietly and modestly in their own way, but we have a
long, long way to go yet.

CHAPTER 3

TENSION IN EVERYDAY LIFE

We all seem to carry unnecessary tension around with us during the day, and sometimes even when we sleep. Occasionally we recognise ourselves as being 'all tensed up' or 'uptight', but most of the time we are unaware of odd parts of our body staying tightened up when it's not necessary.

Though we may not notice the tension, we often feel its effects – headaches, stiffness, aches and pains, indigestion perhaps, or a lack of energy and a general feeling of tiredness, even though there may be difficulty in dropping off at night. How often do we describe our symptoms to the doctor, only to be told 'It's tension. You've got to relax'? 'Easier said than done', you think to yourself as you stomp out of the surgery, with or without a prescription for sedatives, tranquillisers or sleeping tablets.

Many doctors now suggest yoga, relaxation or meditation lessons to their patients, which is a step in the right direction, and I know of classes which include not only patients but the doctors themselves.

DISCOVER YOUR TENSE AREAS

We are all individuals, and learning to recognise our own tension habits is half the battle. To discover some of your own try the following experiment. It only takes five minutes.

Think of how you are sitting *now*, at this very moment. No, don't hurriedly straighten up or uncross your legs (though it may help to check the section on posture afterwards if I've caught you out). Reading a book should be a relaxing activity, but let's see how many areas in your body haven't got the message.

First, think about your eyebrows. Are they pulled together in a frown of concentration? Are your eyes screwed up? (Perhaps you need your glasses checked. Or maybe our print should have been bigger!)

Now, what about your mouth? Are your lips pursed or pulled in a tight line? And your teeth – are they clenched tightly together, making your jaw tense? Your tongue – is it clinging to the roof of the mouth? Pulled back? Hard and narrow instead of full and soft?

By this stage your confidence in your ability to relax may already be waning, and we haven't got below the neck. Don't worry – there is hope. Remember this isn't a competition, there's no score to work out or prizes given for a relaxed jelly or nervous wreck of the week. And after this quiz there are suggestions for putting things right.

Is your chin thrust forward, tensing up your throat and back of the neck? Now the shoulders, a favourite place for tension to wreak havoc: are they pulled up, even ever so slightly, towards the ears? Lift and drop them a few times if you're unsure, and feel the difference.

One of the more subtle ways that we hold tension, in the chest and diaphragm, is detailed in the chapter on breathing (Chapter 15). For the moment just notice whether or not the breath flows freely, gently, easily in and out. When sitting quietly there should be just a gentle rise and fall of the upper abdomen as the breath flows. If you think things are not as they should be, don't worry. Breathing is a bit like walking – if we start thinking about the process in minute detail we seem to lose the knack and are apt to fall over.

Now check your arms. Are they pulled in tight to the body? And the hands, a place tension loves to grip. How tightly are you clutching this book? Do you really need to hold it like that? If one hand is free, what is it doing? Is it tensed, even slightly, into a fist? Or are the fingers stiff and straight or just the thumb poking up in the air? If any of this applies to you, perhaps you'd better let the hands go limp at the wrist and give them a quick shake before continuing.

What about your back? Now you've straightened up (I presume you have) are you sure you're not holding it soldier-stiff or arching the small of the back and pushing the tummy forward? (You can't win, can you?) Thinking about the abdomen, is it pulled in too hard, resisting the gentle rise and fall of the breath?

Now we come to the legs. Are they pulled together tightly, or are they crossed, perhaps with the lower legs and feet wound together?

And lastly, your feet. Like the hands, they are devils for tensing up, and when your feet are unhappy doesn't the rest of the body know it! Are your toes curled tightly, as if to grip the floor? Or are they straight and stiff? Perhaps the big toe alone is poking towards the ceiling. Feet often echo the hands, and vice versa.

A final question. Is anything twitching that shouldn't? Hands fidgeting perhaps, or feet tapping or circling so that they are unable to relax truly. This is a tell-tale sign of tension, even if the rest of the body is still. Even if you don't think you do this, ask a friend or relative – these habits are often the ones that drive others up the wall.

WHY WE SHOULD RELAX

Don't be discouraged if you've found that many or even most of these tension areas apply to you. We all knew instinctively how to relax when we were babies, and our bodies can re-learn, whatever our age or state of health. In fact I have found it easier to teach older students than my teenage daughter who, like most adolescents, was already developing tension habits. You will have developed your own individual pattern of tension over many years, so it may take time to modify it. However the knack of relaxing will return with practice.

Sometimes people are surprised to think that one has to work at relaxation but, as with physical exercise, it usually takes steady practice and patience to improve and to achieve the desired results. Eventually it becomes second nature, with relaxation habits replacing those of tension.

The results of learning to relax are well worth while. When you are tensed up or under stress the whole body is geared for action – heart rate and blood pressure go up, muscles tense, blood flow to the organs and skin is reduced (that's why you go pale). There is also a rise in cortisone level which means, if the tension state is constant, that your immune mechanisms and ability to combat disease are affected – in other words you're more likely to 'go down with something'.

In modern days we rarely explode into the action for which our body tenses us up – fight or flight. It would be rather anti-social to go around thumping people who annoy us or running away from that dreaded interview. So we stay wound up in a state of tension. No wonder then that we end up with all those aches and pains.

However, research has shown that during relaxation the effects of tension can be reversed. Heart rate and blood pressure go down, energy reserves go up, oxygen and cortisone output are reduced and, of course, muscle tension goes down too.

It's nice to know the theory, but even better to discover the practical results yourself. The most obvious one is that at the end of a gentle exercise and relaxation class people often declare that they feel full of energy, even if they could only just make the effort to bring themselves along at the beginning of the class. This feeling of being recharged is common among those who practise yoga. Many older students have also said that practising relaxation helps them to get off to sleep at night without having to rely so much on sleeping tablets. And the very fact that they find they are able to help themselves in such a way boosts their morale and makes for a feeling of increased confidence and well-being.

LEARNING HOW TO RELAX

' All right', you may say, 'I've found some of my tension areas. I'm convinced of the advantages of relaxation. Now what do I do?' Well, you've already made a good start by tuning in to yourself. Awareness is the first, vital step.

Ways of reducing tension

▶ At odd moments during the day, and last thing at night, think through the body as you have just done, searching for any tight areas.
▶ Consciously work on that area, for example lifting and dropping the shoulders, stretching the limbs.
▶ Talk to that part (silently if you don't want heads turning in Sainsbury's). Talk in the gentle way you would soothe a baby: 'Come on now, you don't need to get in that state. Let go . . . relax . . . go soft . . . relax.' Sounds daft, but it works.

▶ Take a deep smooth breath in through the nose and then let out a long and heart-felt sigh. Repeat this two or three times (perhaps only if you're not liable to arouse worried looks).

▶ Practise the 'toe to top' relaxation technique given in Chapter 14 at least once a day – in bed, last thing at night, is a time many people choose.

Any more tension?

The next stage is to indulge in a bit of detective work.

▶ Look carefully at the way you carry out everyday activities – household chores, gardening, eating, etc. Observe yourself and ask questions about the way you do things. For example, 'Do I really need to hold the brush so hard that my knuckles show white? How loosely can I hold it and still control it?'

▶ Try to catch yourself out, checking your posture (bad posture causes a lot of muscular tension). Take a second look at that reflection in the chemist's window. 'Is that slouching individual really me?' Try to think of an invisible thread pulling the top of your head up towards the ceiling and straightening you out.

▶ Photographs will often show up tendencies – perhaps keeping the shoulders lifted. Family and friends can help by pointing out your bad habits (no nagging allowed).

▶ See if you can use the body more evenly. Carry your handbag on the other arm for a change. Try not to stand with the weight always on one hip; do as royalty does and stand with the feet firmly apart, weight equally spread.

▶ If you use a walking aid make sure it is the right height – if in doubt, get it checked. It is common for walking sticks to be too long, with the result that one shoulder is permanently pushed up. The handle should be at hip level.

▶ Make sure that the arms of your favourite chair aren't causing the same effect. Sit with hands in your lap – or change the chair.

▶ Try to work out if there are particular activities that leave you tense in some way. Knitting, for example, may get you in the shoulders, gardening in the back; family visits (though enjoyable) may leave you keyed up. Find movements that will counteract the tension. Stretching is good. Shoulder circling and arm flicking after knitting may help; try a gentle backwards stretch after gardening. Some of these things you will have done instinctively for years. It may help to do the gardening or knitting little and often instead of for long periods at a time or in sudden binges.

▶ Use breathing techniques described in this book. Some tension-releasing breaths may help after the family visit.

Relaxation and exercise

Relaxation goes hand in hand with exercise and after a while you may like to consider the following suggestions.

▶ The body always relaxes better after exercise, even if it's after just a few stretches. Choose a few movements or a complete exercise programme from this book, then do one of the relaxations described.

▶ Don't forget to relax and get your breath in between postures, as well as at the beginning and end of your exercise routine. Think of your body as an elastic band, first stretching, then relaxing.

▶ When doing any exercise (including walking) try and do it in a relaxed way, checking that you're not tightening areas that don't need to come into the action – lifting the shoulder while turning the head for example.

▶ See if you can do some exercise – and relaxation – in a group or with a friend. It will help if you can compare notes, and you will all have a good laugh and benefit from the relaxed atmosphere. Creaking knees may worry you when you practise alone, but when you do knee-bends with friends and find the room resounding to a sound like machine-gun fire it's very reassuring!

Other methods

Other avenues you can explore when trying to deal with unwanted tension are:

▶ Recognise the link between the mind, the emotions and the body – each affects the others. You have probably noticed that if your mind is tensed up, thoughts in turmoil, your body will respond by being tensed, restless and fidgety. We speak of being 'scared stiff' and 'sick with anger'. On the other hand, if we are thinking about a happy event or picturing a soothing scene the body will let go and feel more peaceful.

▶ Use laughter. Give yourself a good dose every day – a TV show, a cartoon book or light reading, family jokes. Let yourself go. Laughter is a great tension releaser and may well be the best medicine.

▶ Use aids which induce relaxation – massage, gentle heat, soothing music, 'relaxation' tapes, stroking the cat, daydreaming, remembering – whatever helps you.

▶ Try cutting down on stimulants such as coffee, cola drinks and (to some extent) tea, particularly if you have trouble sleeping. It's no good doing relaxation or even taking tranquillisers if you are then perking yourself up with frequent, strong coffee. You could try decaffeinated coffee or one of the coffee substitutes. Herbal teas can make a pleasant change once you've found some you like. My mother (a tea addict if ever there was one) has taken to peppermint tea and forty winks after lunch – an excellent combination.

FIRST AID (FOR MOUNTING TENSION OR PANICKY FEELINGS)

Students of all ages found the following STOP technique a useful tool to use in stressful situations. We practised it in class and then, by popular request, it was printed on slips of paper so everyone could keep it in their pocket or bag as a reminder. We are grateful to the late Jane Madders who described the technique, and her family who kindly allow us to reproduce it here.

The STOP Technique
For use when tension and pressure are rising.

▶ Say 'STOP' sharply to yourself (this means stop fussing).
▶ Let your breath go, relaxing your shoulders and hands.
▶ Take in another breath, then let it go – slowly – relaxing your forehead and jaw.
▶ Stay still for a few seconds, then move a little more slowly than before.

▶ If you have to speak, let your voice be a little lower than usual.

As well as the STOP technique, or if a panic attack is threatening, try:

▶ Ten smooth breaths with hands cupped over your nose and mouth.
▶ Press one hand on your forehead and one on the back of your head – or a companion can do this for you.
▶ Put a few drops of Bach Flower Rescue Remedy on your tongue (from chemists or health food stores).

THREE RULES

Finally, there are three rules to bear in mind when you are learning to relax.

Don't feel guilty
Never feel guilty about putting aside time to relax. It is not a self-indulgence. We deserve time to ourselves for re-creation in the true sense of the word. By practising relaxation we will be able to function, and to help others, better. Tell curious friends that it is an important preventative health measure. (It is.)

Be gentle with yourself
Don't be discouraged at the outset if it seems an enormous task that you have taken on. It may help to tackle it in stages and only concentrate on one tension area or habit at a time. It will soon become second nature to you. Then move on to another part. Remember that there are bound to be times when you feel that you aren't getting any better, or are even going backwards. Progress is rarely smooth and constant. The very fact that you are tuning in to yourself so well may mean that you keep discovering things that aren't right. Take heart; see it as a sign of your own increased awareness. Keep in mind that when there is a 'down' it will be followed by an 'up'.

Relax and enjoy this voyage of discovery

CHAPTER 4

THINK UP – GOOD POSTURE

Older people seem to be more aware of their posture than younger generations. Many have told me how Dad used to poke them in the back if they slumped over the table. Some elderly ladies, when they were young, appear to have spent hours walking in circles balancing books on their heads. And there were practices which bordered on torture. Mum-in-law describes how, as a painfully self-conscious adolescent, she was strapped into a special harness which pulled her shoulder-blades together and forced her chest out. It was to no lasting effect, she tells me, except giving her even greater self-consciousness. While not advocating a return to such harsh methods, I do think it is well to consider the importance of *natural* good posture and to work towards the comfort and confidence it brings. You will get more out of your exercises, too, if you don't take bad posture into them.

It's a good idea briefly to check the way you are sitting before starting the exercises, and look at your standing posture before doing any standing movements. The main thing is just to become aware, to tune in to yourself, in the same way as when you are checking for tension. It needn't take long to improve your posture quite radically, and the effort is more mental than physical. A new resident demonstrated this very well. She had already attended one or two exercise classes, and I was looking out for her at the beginning of one of the lessons. You've probably noticed how we recognise people, especially at a distance, more by their familiar posture and way of walking than by their features. Well, I couldn't see this stooped little lady anywhere. I'd walked straight past her, not recognising the upright woman who was really quite tall. She was quite tickled when I told her. She explained 'I was sitting in the class and realised just how stooped and round-shouldered I'd become. I thought to myself "Come on girl, straighten yourself up", and I did!'

THINK UP – WHAT DOES IT MEAN?

The key to good posture, whatever you are doing – sitting, standing or walking – is *think up*. Instead of imagining those books pressing *down* on your head as you walk around, picture the top of your head growing *up* towards the sky. Imagine an invisible string coming from the crown of your head and being gently pulled towards the ceiling. You can get the right feeling by grasping a lock of hair at the top of your head and pulling it gently upwards. If there's nothing there to grasp – sorry fellas – you'll just have to make good use of your imagination. Try bringing this feeling to mind at odd times during the day. Don't stiffen up, though, like a toy soldier: just feel a gentle lengthening right up through the spine, from the base up to where the neck joins the head.

This lengthening has many beneficial effects. Not only do you look better and your clothes hang well, but, more importantly, everything inside your body has more room and can function better. We all know that bad posture can cause muscular aches and pains, but if your back is slumped and your shoulders rounded your stomach and lungs are being squashed up, making it harder for them to work well. It can even mean that you are more likely to get chest infections and indigestion. There are psychological benefits too – lifting your body gives the spirits a lift.

Of course, the spine is meant to have gentle curves, but we have to be careful not to exaggerate them (which is the commonest fault) or go to the other extreme and try to flatten them out completely.

Apparently we are slightly shorter by night-time than when we are awake. During the day spinal discs compress. Blame gravity, but some occupations aggravate this tendency: I was once offered a job as a human cannonball – I imagined the roar of the crowd, the breathtaking flight – but I declined. It would take an awful lot of stretching and posture work to counteract the impact of landing!

Here is a guide to checking your posture when standing and sitting and while moving generally. It doesn't take as long as you might think, and briefly going through the checklist in your head can quickly become a habit.

STANDING

Feet

Look at your feet. They should be slightly, or hip-width, apart and parallel, like tram lines. Sitting, standing or walking, this is the way they are designed to be used. Keep an eye on them – they have a mind of their own and don't give up old habits easily. Bad placing of the feet can give rise to problems in the knees, hips and back. Feel the weight going evenly through both feet, so you are well balanced.

Knees

These should not be locked back, but should be ever so slightly bent.

Hips

Your weight should go evenly through both hips, so it isn't all to one side. Your 'tail' should be tucked under slightly, so there isn't a big hollow in the small of the back. Women often have this tendency, aided and abetted by high heels. If you do stand like this, then there is more likely to be low backache and muscular weakness there.

Tummy

This can be slightly pulled in (remember to keep breathing, though) so you are using your own muscular 'corset' and not relying on underwear manufacturers for support. Ladies – never mind about burning your bra, it's the corsets which should go up in smoke!

Chest

It should feel open and free, neither caved in nor thrust aggressively forward. Feel both front and back of the chest equally broad. You can help by pulling the shoulder blades gently towards each other, then letting them relax, but not slump.

Shoulders

If you have checked your chest correctly, the shoulders should not be rounded. See that they aren't pulled up towards the ears either – this is very common, especially when you are tense or cold. Let the shoulders relax down away from the ears so your neck is long. Lift and drop the shoulders a few times if it helps.

Arms

Let your arms hang loose by your sides. Palms should be against the outside of the thighs, ideally the tip of the middle finger in line with the side seam of your trousers or skirt. If this isn't the case don't force them into the 'correct' position, just picture them coming nearer to it. Look for any tendency to stand or walk with the arms turned, palms facing behind you, as this can cause or aggravate shoulder problems.

Neck

Keep picturing that invisible string pulling gently on the crown of your head, and your neck should lengthen so there is no arch in the back of it. Tucking the chin in slightly will help. Some people try to stand tall by pushing the chin upwards or forwards. This will merely compress the neck and shorten it – no help at all. Check the back of your neck with your hand if you're unsure.

SITTING

The checklist for a good sitting posture is basically the same as when standing.

First, wriggle your bottom as far back as you can into the chair. This applies wherever you are sitting – in the car, armchair, dining chair, anywhere. If your legs don't quite reach the floor and are dangling unsupported you really need a cushion or some other support under them. Check that you are not sitting on your 'tail bone', but that the weight is going squarely and equally through both sitting bones. Keep the back straight but not stiff; don't let it hollow as you endeavour to sit up well.

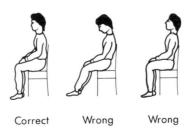

Correct   Wrong   Wrong

All this takes a little thought at first, but soon becomes routine. If you sit in an armchair, especially for long periods of time, see that the arms of the chair aren't so high that they force your shoulders up, making them and your neck tight and aching. A yoga teacher once visited a residential home for the elderly and was puzzled to find so many residents with aches and pains in their necks and shoulders. She found the armchairs to be the source of the problem and there was relief all round when they discovered that resting the hands in the lap instead of on the chair-arms was the answer.

ON THE MOVE

Sitting down, the elegant and safe way
Step backwards so that you can feel the back of your legs touching the seat. If the chair has projecting arms take hold of these and leaning forward a little let them take some of your weight while you slowly lower yourself into the seat.

Getting up again
Come towards the front of your chair holding its arms if it has them, if not then grip the front corners of the seat. Now put your heels well back under your chair, gradually leaning forward so that you can feel your weight going down over your feet. Then stand up by pushing with the arms and at the same time straightening the knees with those powerful thigh muscles. You should stand for a moment or two, still holding the arms of the chair, so you find your balance before moving away. This method is worth cultivating as you won't need to lurch too far forward and it can also strengthen your legs.

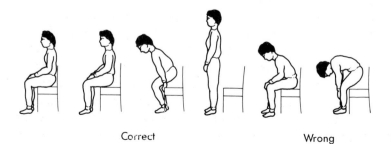

Correct   Wrong

Walking

Try to keep that tall feeling when walking; let the hips and arms swing freely, enjoying the sense of motion and not stiffening up. You may not find this so easy if you use a walking stick or other such aid, but the same principle applies.

Bending

Most people know this, but it is worth repeating because it is so important. When you are lifting *bend the knees*. Similarly when you are working in the garden, cleaning floors, making beds or performing other such tasks, try squatting or kneeling instead of stooping.

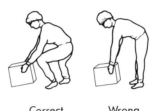

Correct   Wrong

THE IMPORTANCE OF GOOD POSTURE

It is well worth the slight effort needed to cultivate better posture. Even the oldest and most disabled people taking part in our exercise groups have shown that they can quickly respond to suggestions for improving their posture. Don't be disheartened if you have health problems that make your spine other than the ideal shape; we aren't aiming for the perfect body, just one that is a little straighter and more comfortable.

Perhaps you feel that your general size or shape leaves a lot to be desired. Many of us have a 'thing' about one or more parts of ourselves. Short, dark and skinny, I spent much of my life longing to be tall and elegant. Yoga teaches us to be comfortable with what we've been given. After all, if it can't be changed, why waste energy worrying over it? No matter what your size or figure, be proud of it. It is you. Why should you conform to other people's ideas as to what is ideal? Marvel at the diversity of nature. Accept yourself as part of it.

Remember the words of the song, 'Walk tall, walk straight and look the world right in the eye' – do just that.

GADGETS TO HELP

If you find retrieving objects from the floor a real problem, there are gadgets designed to help with this. Have you noticed how when your body refuses to bend in the middle, everyday objects develop a life of their own and the floor a magnetic attraction? Things leap out of your hands at every available opportunity. I learnt this for a fact during the last few weeks of pregnancy. My 90-year-old students were more agile than me and I would have dearly loved a loan of one of their 'grabbers'.

And what about other problems which come about when there is restricted movement or strength? If, for example, your toilet seat is too low or it is a struggle to get out of the bath alone, talk to your doctor or community nurse about it. There are simple aids available (often free from the Social Services or the Red Cross) which can make life much easier and help to conserve your energy, dignity and independence. National and local organisations set up to help sufferers of particular conditions may also provide very practical advice. See Useful Addresses page 158.

It is most important, to make sure your walking aid is the right one for you at this moment. There may be ups and downs caused by stiffness, accidents or illness which mean that you need a tripod or wheeled aid for a time before returning to your usual walking stick. I know of many elderly friends who have done this. It's good to be adaptable.

It is also very helpful to have not only the right aid at the right time but also to have it at the correct height for you. The walking stick handle should be at the same height as your hip joint. Ask your doctor or community nurse to help assess your needs, and have the equipment adjusted if necessary. Also be sure that you know exactly how to walk with it – even using a walking stick needs a system and you'd be surprised how many folk I've seen moving around, happily carrying their walking frame! To avoid accidents have the rubber stoppers on the end of your stick or aid regularly checked and renewed. They can wear out surprisingly quickly, particularly the old-fashioned black ones.

And there's no need to feel that you're giving in if you resort to a walking aid. I've seen them give people a new lease of life. It can mean that you're independent again – instead of having to depend on someone proffering their arm all the time. These aids can give you your confidence back and make you feel safer too. There are some novel aids around now which have all sorts of advantages, including one that looks like a small version of a supermarket trolley; as well as being useful round the house it is the envy of many weary shoppers on their way to and from the corner store.

CHAPTER 5

BEFORE YOU START

Before you launch into these simple exercises just take a few moments to consider some practical points. No special equipment or clothing is needed, and the advice that follows is really plain common sense. If there are other folk in the vicinity, it's as well to prepare the ground in advance, especially if there is a group of you or you are practising in an unfamiliar room or hall. Let people know that you will need peace and quiet, and privacy – strictly no observers – unless they join in!

ROOM

Make sure there will be enough space around your chair for you to lift your arms and legs without knocking the furniture (or friends). The room should be comfortably warm, not stuffy, with some fresh air if possible, but no draughts.

CHAIR

A firm straight-backed chair is best – a kitchen or dining chair is fine. Sit well back in the chair and see if your feet are still firmly on the floor. If not, place a cushion or other support beneath them.

If you have to stay sitting in an armchair or wheelchair you too should wriggle your bottom into the back of the chair, your spine straight and well supported, arranging cushions to help if necessary. This will help your posture, making the exercises easier and more beneficial. You may need a cushion beneath the feet too. Some folk like to retire to a nearby armchair for the final relaxation – this is quite all right as long as you don't allow yourself to slump into it.

CLOTHING

Any loose comfy clothing will do. If you possess one, a tracksuit is ideal, but women can manage very well in a comfortable dress or skirt.

Nothing tight should be worn. Belts, collars, even foundation garments, can constrict and restrict. Give your feet a treat – remove your shoes and socks, tights or stockings, if possible.

PROPS

The basic programme outlined at the beginning of Appendix 1, and the majority of other sessions, require no special props. Occasionally a scarf or belt will come in handy, sometimes an extra chair – such items will be mentioned at the start of a programme.

A cassette or record player is also useful. Many people find they relax better when there is soothing music in the background. Keep a recording of your favourite piece to hand, or perhaps you might invest in a special relaxation tape. Have these within easy reach so you can switch on and relax at the end of your exertions.

MOST IMPORTANTLY

Keep all movements *slow and smooth*, rather like working in slow motion. If you are getting breathless, huffing and puffing, this means that you are working too fast or trying too hard, so slow down and find the right pace for *you*.

No competition

There is no competition with other people or yourself. We are all quite different and need to work in different ways. Listen to your own body. You will find that it will vary from day to day, even from hour to hour. If you are part of a group and you have a show-off in your midst, remember the tale of the hare and the tortoise; don't be tempted to compete with them.

No strain

Try and find the fine line between effort and strain. If a particular movement is uncomfortable or just doesn't feel right for you – don't do it. If you have limitations due to illness or injury don't force movement, but take it as far as it will go without strain or pain. For example, if you have a stiff shoulder that hurts if you try to lift the whole arm right up to the ear, only raise it as high as shoulder level if that's all right – never mind what other people can do. It's not what you do, it's the way that you do it.

Stop immediately if you have:

▶ pain
▶ dizziness
▶ feelings of sickness or being unwell
▶ unusual tiredness

It might be that you've just overdone things a bit, but if such symptoms continue see your doctor.

Start gradually

Take your time to find how much exercise at a time is right for you. Better to start gently, using just stretches and warm ups, and then go on to as much of the basic programme in Appendix 1 as you feel happy with. It's like testing the water with your toes rather than diving straight in. Gradually you will find you can include a greater variety and perhaps some more demanding postures.

A few minutes a day is often better than a full 30–40-minute session once a week. In my experience most older people find 20–30 minutes of exercises quite enough at a time. After the relaxation which follows you should feel revived and energetic (if perhaps a little dreamy). If you feel worn out then the session has been too long or ambitious, and you'll need to modify it.

All the suggested programmes in Appendix 1 are designed to fit into 30 or 40 minutes, including relaxation periods at the beginning and end of the session and short breathers in between postures.

Relaxation

Don't forget about relaxation. It's sometimes a temptation to leave it out when you are practising alone or are short of time. As in conventional yoga, it is important always to start with a short period of relaxation and finish with a longer one.

Keep breathing

Gradually try to work with the breath, but don't worry if this takes time. If you find it's as much as you can do to follow the movements, concentrate on them and just let the breath flow naturally. But do remember, *keep* breathing. It's surprising how often we hold our breath when concentrating.

MEDICAL CONSIDERATIONS

Just as younger yoga students are advised to seek their doctor's approval before starting lessons, so it is important that older students too should put their doctor in the picture. As I said in the preface, it may be as well to take along this book, as his or her idea of exercise or yoga may be something quite different from the reality. If the doctor gets the mistaken idea that you are going to run a marathon, stand on your head or tie yourself in knots, it's not surprising if the answer will be a horrified 'No'. However most doctors are glad to see elderly patients keen to keep moving, especially with a suitable exercise regime.

If you have specific medical problems certain movements may not be helpful and will be better omitted or modified. Your doctor should advise you on these, and some suggestions are made below. But don't be put off if you have a medical condition or are not 100 per cent fit. The movements in our programmes are so slow and smooth that you will have plenty of time to feel your way into them, and you will be able to stop if you sense something is not going to be right for you.

The following notes, regarding some of the commonest health problems in elderly people, may be useful.

Arthritis

Arthritis seems to be a common complaint in older people. The dictionary definition of arthritis is 'inflammation of a joint', and it can be long-standing (chronic) or sudden and short (acute). There are two main types – rheumatoid arthritis and osteoarthritis. You may already know which type you have.

Osteoarthritis is a degeneration (a wearing out) of the bones. It tends to be chronic and involves mainly weight-bearing joints such as hips, knees, etc. The joint surface deteriorates and the result is pain and restricted movement. If your condition is only mild the gentle exercises given in this book, if practised regularly, can be of very real benefit. And if the circulation to, and the muscles around, the joint are improved by the exercises, the joint will be strengthened too. I have seen quite dramatic improvements. If your arthritis is more advanced there may be joint changes that cannot be reversed. In this case do what movements you can within the limits set by pain. Even if stiff hips and knees are a problem, working on keeping the spine flexible will be of general help, and the exercises may actually keep the arthritis in check.

Rheumatoid arthritis is a general illness, affecting not only the joints (most usually the smaller ones – fingers, wrists and knees may become fixed) but the whole system. It is usually chronic, with flare-ups at varying intervals, during which the person feels generally unwell with accompanying pain in the joints. Although the emphasis in all arthritic conditions is on keeping moving, during an acute attack it is better to do only breathing exercises and relaxation and to rest, rather than to push yourself physically. A joint must *never* ever be worked while it is inflamed. When the acute stage has passed and inflammation has 'burnt out', gentle exercise can be resumed, though you must carefully observe the usual guidelines and work without strain. With osteoarthritis it is acceptable to work through a little pain to get stiff joints moving again, but this is *not* the case with rheumatoid arthritis.

If your knees are affected it will be better to use sitting or lying postures rather than standing ones. Such postures will allow a wider range of movement and there will be less strain. Not surprisingly, rheumatoid arthritis causes much tension and tiredness so the relaxation and breathing exercises are particularly helpful.

Spinal problems
Gentle exercise can bring greater ease of movement and increased suppleness in the spine, whether the trouble is due to arthritis, a past

'slipped disc' (actual or presumed), or general muscular stiffness. Slow gentle stretching movements done once or twice daily can give real benefit, as can improving general posture (see the section which deals with the back, beginning on page 61). Make sure the room, and your back in particular, are nice and warm to start with and always remember to do warm-up movements before more vigorous exercise. If there is general stiffness when you wake in the morning, have a good stretch within the warmth of your bed before getting up.

However, if your back trouble has been diagnosed as ankylosing spondylitis be very cautious when exercising. Similarly, if you know your bones have become fragile (as in severe osteoporosis), arm and leg movements may be all that is advisable – as well as breathing and relaxation, of course.

Heart trouble

Exercise can help and strengthen the heart, although it must be of the right sort in the right quantity. Many people with heart disease use, enjoy and benefit from our yoga sessions, but you must bear in mind earlier advice and modify movements, slowing them down, cutting down on repeats and resting if you feel breathless or uncomfortable. Your most important rule is to be guided by your breath.

If you have congestive heart failure and are always breathless, do only exercises with minimal movement – hands and feet, eye exercises, etc. – and work on the simplest breathing exercises. Relaxation and visualisation come into their own here.

If you have suffered a heart attack (coronary thrombosis) you will have had special or intensive care in hospital after it first happened. This may have left you feeling quite frightened of moving about or taking the gentlest exercise, even when you are well recovered. However, as you recover and a scar forms in the damaged heart muscle you will be advised that you can gradually get moving again. The coronary circulation will improve and your heart muscle will then strengthen as it is stimulated by gradual exercise. Be guided by your medical advisers and by your own body's response. It is probably a good idea to spend several sessions practising just the breath of relaxation (see Chapter 15 on breathing) before adding movements – action breaths. This will help to overcome tension in the chest and shoulders and increase your confidence. There are plenty of nonstrenuous exercises detailed in this book, many not even as strenuous as walking, so although you may be rather worried about moving at first, you can feel your way gradually back to sensible exercise.

The same applies if you have angina. Many of our elderly students may have degrees of angina but still take part and benefit from the exercise sessions, just taking care not to attempt things that produce chest pain.

Students with a heart condition or breathlessness will probably prefer not to do much with the arms lifted or held high. When doing 'mountain breaths', for example, you may be happier keeping your fingertips on your shoulders and just raising and lowering your elbows. You will see other modifications to choose from among the various exercises and postures detailed in Chapters 6 to 11.

And it is probably a good idea to read the following advice about blood pressure, too.

High and low blood pressure

If you have high blood pressure you will probably prefer not to take your head too low in forward bends, etc. When straightening up keep the chin tucked in, lifting the head last. This helps stop you feeling dizzy (and applies to students of all ages). Relaxation and breathing exercises can be very helpful for those with high blood pressure. You shouldn't do any breath holding, though, and this is one reason why no such exercises are included in this book. Do check that you don't have the habit of holding the breath while concentrating on exercises.

Have you read Chapter 3, on tension in everyday life? Lessening general tenseness should help control high blood pressure, as will going easy with the salt-cellar – make the hole in the top of it smaller, or better still try one of the new low-sodium table-salts now available. Such self-help remedies can't do you any harm, and may well do some good.

As we get older, even when there is no blood pressure problem, it takes longer for our circulation to adjust from a lying position to a sitting one and from a sitting to a standing one. This is why we get dizzy if we rise too quickly, often noticed when sitting up and getting out of bed in the morning. All such movements should therefore be done slowly, with thought, and in gradual stages if necessary. This applies even more if you know you have low blood pressure.

Strokes

Simple poses and exercises are particularly valuable for the person recovering from a stroke. You may be rather nervous at first, especially where balance is concerned. Don't worry – you can start off doing many of the exercises in an armchair or wheelchair. A limb which has lost its power can be lifted, by using the good limb to raise it, by using a strap or even by pulling on the trouser leg to help it up, or by having a sympathetic person to put the limb through the movement for you. Don't let them pull you around too much, though – slowly does it.

Tremor

If you have a tremor, leave out the warm ups, etc., that direct you to shake or flap your hands or feet.

IN CONCLUSION

I could go into a great amount of detail listing different ailments and their relevance when exercising. However, it is not the intention to make this a medical encyclopaedia. If you use your common sense and sensitivity you will come to no harm from gentle exercise. It is still safer to exercise carefully than to do nothing at all.

Having read this far you should be well prepared and itching to start. You can either plunge into the next few chapters, on the various postures and variations, or, alternatively, if you want to take things more easily, try the basic programme at the beginning of Appendix 1.

The only advice that remains is: Relax and enjoy it.

CHAPTER 6

How to Start

However short your practice session always start and end with relaxation. Always warm up. *Don't* strain; just go as far as you can and stop. Adapt postures to your own limitations. Relax and let your breath return to normal between postures.

ACTION BREATHS

At the start of a practice use action breaths as described below (or in the basic programme on page 137. These not only give you a stretch but the accompanying deep breaths wake you up and bring in more oxygen, preparing the body for movement – good to do first thing in the morning. They can be done seated or standing.

Mountain breaths
Deep smooth breaths in time with arm movements. Repeat two or more times. If you prefer, place fingertips on shoulders lifting elbows as you breathe in and lowering as you breathe out.

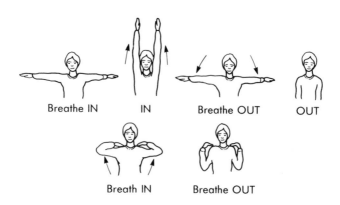

Breathe IN   IN   Breathe OUT   OUT

Breath IN   Breathe OUT

▶ Same movement, but with the arms lifted forwards. Do three or six times.
▶ Fingertips on shoulders, lifting elbows as you breathe in, circling elbows towards each other as you breathe out. Do three or six times.

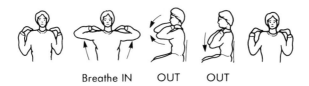

Breathe IN   OUT   OUT

Swimming in space

This movement helps you to feel the breath rising from the tummy, through the rib cage, right to the top of the chest as you breathe in, and empty all the way down as you breathe out.

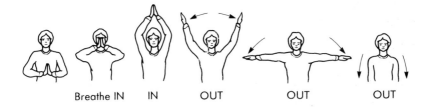

Breathe IN   IN   OUT   OUT   OUT

WARM-UPS

Whatever the weather, it's best to warm up (or rather loosen up) before starting to exercise. As well as the shaking and flicking exercises on page 138 described in the basic programme, the following ideas really get the circulation going – especially useful in cold weather.

▶ Make your hands into relaxed fists and gently thump your body all over, from head to feet. Don't thump on varicose veins.
▶ Rub your body in the same way; pinch your 'spare tyre' round your middle.

And here are some more general warming-up movements. They should leave your hands and feet tingling.

- ▶ Flick wrists as if shaking off drops of water.
- ▶ Take fingertips to shoulders, then flick arms straight.
- ▶ Lean forward, letting arms hang limp and heavy. Shake and wriggle arms and shoulders, feeling them really loose. Straighten up slowly.
- ▶ Lift alternate knees as if pedalling.
- ▶ Pat thighs rapidly with hands.
- ▶ Stamp feet rapidly on floor.
- ▶ Pat your thighs and stamp your feet together (it'll sound as if the cavalry's coming.)
- ▶ Get your breath back.

STRETCHES

We often indulge in a good stretch after a period of relaxation, sleep or just sitting still for a while. Our bodies instinctively do it to release tension and get moving. It is a natural start to any period of exercise and if you are short on time or energy just using these stretches (preferably after some action breaths and a warm-up) may be enough to set you up for the day or to ease off at night.

- ▶ You could start by stretching just one arm or leg at a time.

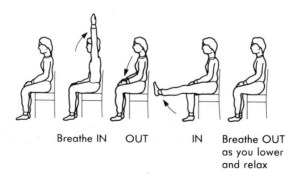

Breathe IN   OUT   IN   Breathe OUT
as you lower
and relax

▶ Stretch through one side of the body, then the other. . .

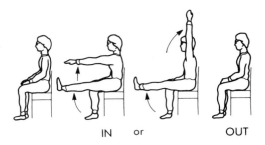

IN   or   OUT

▶ then diagonally. . .

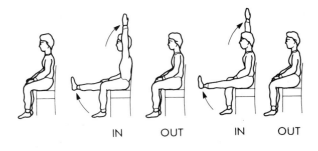

IN   OUT   IN   OUT

▶ then right through.

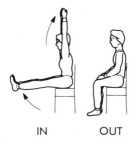

IN   OUT

Picking grapes off the ceiling

This involves stretching with one arm towards the ceiling, then with the other arm. Keep it going four or six times, trying not to sway from side to side. Then breathe out and lower your arms, and wriggle your shoulders to ease them.

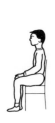

Breathing IN lift both arms close to ears	OUT Pause, soften	IN Stretch towards ceiling with one arm	OUT Pause here	IN Stretch other arm

▶ A less tiring variation on picking grapes is to rest one hand on the head while the other stretches.

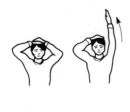

Breathe IN lifting arms to shoulder height	Let breath flow naturally, stretch forward with each arm in turn

Pulling in the rope

This can be done as well as or instead of picking grapes. The idea is to stretch forward with each arm in turn, as if pulling in a rope

The four-way stretch

The idea here is to bend first to one side, then to the other, and then to bend first backwards and then forwards. It can be done seated or standing, with hands on the hips, hands on a chair to help balance, or with hands linked and held overhead if you want a really strong stretch and are sure of your balance.

When standing, feet can be hip-width apart, really wide or close together. Or try the same stretches with the feet in these three positions in turn – feel the subtle difference to the movement. And remember to keep your back straight from the hips on these standing forward bends.

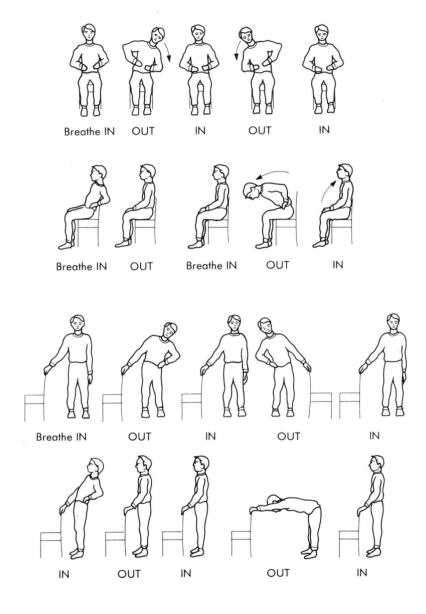

Breathe IN   OUT   IN   OUT   IN

Breathe IN   OUT   Breathe IN   OUT   IN

Breathe IN   OUT   IN   OUT   IN

IN   OUT   IN   OUT   IN

The breathing rule is to breathe out as you bend and breathe in as you straighten. However, if you can't fit the breathing in at first, just concentrate on the movements – but keep breathing!

WHAT NEXT?

In the following chapters are a series of movements and postures for the various parts of your body, starting with your head and going down to your toes.

You can choose a selection of these if you want, and build them up into your own personal programme, as explained in Appendix 1. Alternatively, if you have a particular problem, e.g. stiff hands or tight hips, you could try some of the appropriate movements at odd times during the day. But don't attempt all the suggestions for that area in one session – it might prove to be too much, making you very tired at the time and painfully stiff afterwards. However, a little stiffness may be expected when you are working muscles that are out of the habit of being used.

CHAPTER 7

THE HEAD AND NECK

SCALP

This can feel tight sometimes. A little massage can stimulate circulation here and may help if you feel 'headachey'. You can do it yourself or take turns with a partner.

Scalp massage
Place your fingertips firmly on your head. Make circular movements with the fingers, not brushing over the hair but making the scalp really wriggle under the fingers. It may look as if your hair has become a wig which is shifting round on your head.

Gradually work in this way all over the head. Your scalp may feel very tender in places; this is quite normal, but go a little easier in these spots.

Hair tweaking
(I'm afraid this is only possible if you still sport a 'crowning glory'.)

Hold a small bunch of hair firmly between your fingertips, close to its roots. Then slide your fingers to the ends of the hair in jerky little tugs. Work all over the head in this way.

The resulting spiky halo may look a little weird, but the warm tingle is lovely.

FOREHEAD

▶ Lift and drop eyebrows (as in the basic programme on page 137).
▶ Place fingertips lightly in the centre of the forehead.
▶ Stroke smoothly across to the temples.

▶ Make small firm circular movements on the temples.
▶ Lift fingers back to the centre of the forehead and repeat several times.

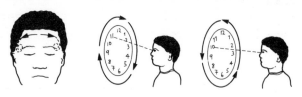

EYE EXERCISES

The following exercises can help to strengthen the muscles round the eyes. They are good to do after a spell of reading, knitting or watching television.

Looking round the clock

Keep your head completely still while doing this. Only the eyeballs should move. Blink whenever you need. And don't forget to remove your spectacles first.

▶ Imagine a clock in front of your face.
▶ Look clockwise at each number in turn.
▶ Then look anticlockwise.
▶ Blink rapidly, relax and palm eyes (see next page).
▶ In the same way, look up and down your clock, then side to side, then repeat in the opposite order.
▶ Blink, relax and palm eyes.

Changing focus

▶ Holding a pointed finger in front of your face (about 1 foot away).
▶ Focus your gaze on the fingertip.
▶ Focus your gaze on the background behind the finger.
▶ Repeat this several times.
▶ Blink, relax and palm eyes.

Palming eyes

This is nice and soothing. Always finish eye exercises with it.

- ▶ Gently close your eyes.
- ▶ Rub the palms of your hands together.
- ▶ Place the palms lightly over the eyes.
- ▶ Leave them there for half a minute or more.
- ▶ Open your eyes within your hands.
- ▶ Gradually let more light in, giving your eyes time to adjust as the hands are slowly lifted away.

JAW AND MOUTH

We hold tension in this area by keeping the jaws clamped together, and by gritting or grinding the teeth – often done while we sleep. The result may be aching round the teeth, in the jaw, in the face, even in the neck and head. Such tension and pain may be caused by your bite, too; by the way your teeth or dentures mesh together. Ask your dentist to check your occlusion (bite). Any adjustment to your teeth or dentures is usually very easy to make and the results can be very effective. My dentist tells of chronic neuralgia and migraine sufferers who have gained relief in this way.

Jaw exercises

- ▶ Clench your teeth together; feel the tension in your face.
- ▶ Let your teeth part and the jaw relax.
- ▶ Open your mouth and jut your jaw forward; then relax.
- ▶ With lips parted, move your lower jaw in a circle, first one way then the other.
- ▶ **Silent scream** – open your mouth really wide, then let it relax.

Tension check

If you find that you tend to clench your jaw, check it at odd times of day. Try to correct the habit by consciously relaxing the jaw. This doesn't mean that you have to walk around with the jaw hanging open, flycatching. Say to yourself 'Teeth parted, lips together.'

WHOLE FACE

▶ Screw your whole face up tightly.
▶ Slowly let it smooth out completely – picture the wrinkles and laughter lines melting away.
▶ Repeat a few times.

This is always good for a laugh when done in company. All these facial exercises are said to be beautifying, so keep practising in hope.

NECK AND HEAD

Chicken neck
Sit upright, then stretch the neck forward, pointing the chin out and back again, like a chicken. Make sure you finish with your chin back!

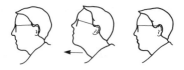

Daily neck movements
The following sequence will encourage or keep the full range of movement in the neck. Remember to do them slowly, smoothly and to hold the position (but not the breath) for a few moments.

▶ Sit tall. Move the chin slowly down towards your chest. Pause, and feel the weight of the head helping the neck to lengthen. Then slowly lift the head straight.

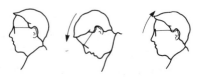

▶ Keeping the rest of the body still, put the head on one side, ear moving down towards shoulder. Don't let the shoulder pull up –

that's cheating. Slowly straighten the head. Then repeat to the other side.

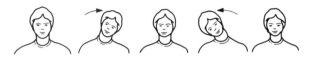

▶ Slowly turn the head to look over one shoulder as far as it will comfortably go. Pause, keeping the shoulders relaxed. Turn the head back to the centre. Then repeat to the other side.

▶ **Pendulum movement** – start with your chin towards your chest. Circle your chin across your chest to look over your right shoulder. Then make a big semi-circle across your chest to look over your left shoulder. Aim to keep a smooth movement going as you make the semi-circles across your chest.

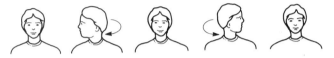

Chin towards chest   Circle chin across chest to look over right shoulder   Make big semi-circle across chest to look over left shoulder

HEAD ROLLING – A WARNING

Some like to roll the head in a full circle, taking it right back so that the chin is up towards the ceiling. For those who have problems in the neck this is *not* recommended. Strong arching of the neck is a strain, even when done very slowly, and the head is surprisingly heavy. For the older age-group in general I think it is preferable to use just the pendulum movement instead.

CHAPTER 8

SHOULDERS AND ARMS

ARM MOVEMENTS

Swinging arms

These can be done as warm ups, sitting or standing. Keep the movements loose and free.

- ▶ Bend from the waist. Let the arms hang limp.
- ▶ Shake your arms and shoulders, loose and heavy.
- ▶ Swing both arms by your sides, forward and back.
- ▶ Scissor your arms back and forth across the front of your body.
- ▶ Tuck your chin in and unroll to an upright position very slowly.

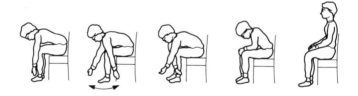

Circling arms – windmill

- ▶ Circle one arm slowly forwards, then backwards.
- ▶ Then circle the other arm.
- ▶ Now circle both together.

If the above movement is too strong, try circling the elbow with your fingertips on your shoulder as a variation.

Rotating arms

▶ Let your arms hang loose by your sides.
▶ Rotate your arms so the palms and inner arms face forwards.
▶ Rotate them so the backs of the hands and arms are to the front.
▶ Finish by returning your arms to their natural position by the sides.

Breathe IN   Breathe OUT

Be careful

If you have one arm with weakness or limited movement (due to stroke, injury, or a 'frozen shoulder' perhaps) use the good arm to help the weaker one through its range of movements. For example, rest the hand of the weaker arm on top of the good one; lift together as far as possible, then lower together.

Be guided by any pain. Don't force the arm, but picture it moving easily in your mind's eye as you do such movements. A partner can help you by moving the weaker arm for you, but make sure that they know what they're doing and don't let them get over-enthusiastic, moving too far, too fast or too jerkily. Be sure that *you* are in control and let them know if they're not doing it right, or if it hurts.

SEQUENCES

Choose only *one* of the following sequences (with the exception, perhaps, of elephant ears). Repeat each of them about three times, and afterwards release any tension in the shoulders by rotating them and lifting and dropping them. And *remember*, keep the movements slow and smooth, work with the breath when possible and, above all, don't strain. All these may be done seated.

Swimming

This is like breast-stroke. Bring your arms up to the side, swing forward and pull into the chest. Now reverse – push forward, to the side and down.

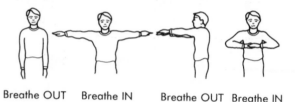

Breathe OUT   Breathe IN   Breathe OUT   Breathe IN

Elephant ears

Link your fingers behind your ears, move your elbows towards each other, then move them back, pulling your shoulder blades towards each other.

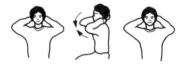

▶ Link fingers with your arms in front of you, palms towards you, then repeat with the palms away from you. Then repeat the movement with your arms behind you. Now loosen your shoulders by rotating them and lifting and dropping them, keeping your arms down.

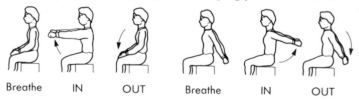

Breathe   IN   OUT   Breathe   IN   OUT

Hornpipe

Place one arm across the front of your waist and the other across the back, then reverse the movement smoothly and slowly.

Cow head

Raise one arm, bend it at the elbow and let the hand fall down behind your shoulders. Now bend the other arm, put the hand up behind the back in a 'half-nelson' and try to reach the other hand. Holding a scarf may help. Repeat on the other side. Now loosen your shoulders and relax.

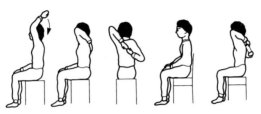

Another swimming movement

This works on your shoulders and arms, as well as helping to open the chest and benefit the lungs. It is good to practise if you have a tendency to round shoulders.

- ▶ Hands in prayer position on the chest.
- ▶ Stretch the arms forward as if about to dive.
- ▶ Swoop arms round in a breast-stroke movement, and link hands behind your back.
- ▶ Let shoulders and arms relax, then lift arms only.
- ▶ Bend forward, tummy towards thighs, back and neck straight.
- ▶ Slowly straighten up.
- ▶ Release your arms and wriggle your shoulders to ease them.

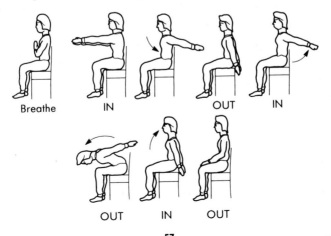

SOME EASIER MOVEMENTS

Directing traffic

▶ Lift arms forward to shoulder height.
▶ Stretch arms to one side without turning trunk.
▶ Move your arms back to the middle again (first position).
▶ Take arms to other side and repeat.

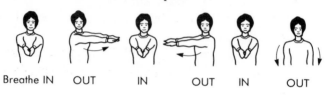

Breathe IN   OUT   IN   OUT   IN   OUT

Elbow snaps

This is not as violent as it sounds. It is rather like punching or rowing, but instead of the feeling of pushing your fists forwards, concentrate on straightening the elbows.

▶ Form your hands into fists, thumbs outside, pointing down.
▶ Then put the back of each fist towards your chest; elbows should be bent and the fists about 4 inches apart.
▶ Straighten your arms, bringing your elbows towards each other. As you do this the back of your fists should turn towards the ceiling.

Keep the movement slow and smooth at first. When you become more used to it you can speed it up, doing six snaps in all. No special breathing pattern is required.

As a variation you can hold your arms lower if your shoulders feel strained.

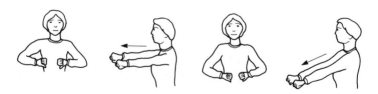

HAND AND FINGER EXERCISES

Rub your hands and fingers first. Then choose just one or two exercises at a time.

- ► Use one hand to press each finger of the other towards the palm. Press the tip, middle and lower part of each finger (and thumb). Press between, not on, joints.
- ► Press each finger backwards in the same way.
- ► Grasp all the fingers in the other hand, press gently back, then repeat with the other hand.
- ► Try to make a fan effect by crossing each finger over the next.
- ► Let the hands flop, then shake them hard – as in playing the piano then juggling.

Starfish

- ► Place the fingertips on your lap or on a table.
- ► Press the fingers slowly out into a star shape.

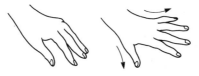

Casting a spell
This is a good one.

- ► Make the hands into fists, with the backs of your hands close to your shoulders.
- ► Push your arms strongly forwards, spreading the fingers wide.

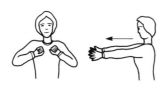

WRISTS

Inner wrist stretch

This is a hard one.

▶ Place your fingertips, palms facing forwards, on your thighs or on a surface next to your hips.

▶ Endeavour to straighten your elbows and place your palms flat on your thighs or on the surface.

This is difficult, so don't push hard.

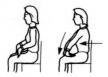

Queenly wave

Support your elbow on the arm of a chair or in the free hand. Make a circle with the hand, first one way then the other.

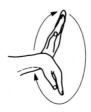

CHAPTER 9

THE BACK

There is a saying that 'You are as young as your spine', and this does seem to be true. Anyone who has put their back out will testify that it can feel as if they've aged 50 years overnight. If the spine is stiff or painful it hampers normal body movement and can affect the functioning of internal organs too, so it is definitely in our interests to keep our backs as supple and free-moving as possible.

So many people – young and old alike – have problems with their backs that this is now a common reason for their taking up yoga. Stretching gently and smoothly, taking the spine through its natural range of movements, can gradually ease and strengthen the back muscles. Swimming, dancing and other forms of gentle exercise are also to be recommended. I even heard of a man who had suffered with rheumatics in his back for years describing the marvellous relief he enjoyed after he took up bell-ringing.

BACK PAIN

I presume that if you suffer with chronic back pain you will have had it checked out by your doctor. Sometimes the cause may not be directly related to the spine at all. Soft tissue conditions can be a cause of nagging backache – for example prolapse of the womb.

Whether the cause of back pain is muscular, rheumatic, or you have 'put it out', *don't* do exercises while the pain is really bad. This is very important. Instead you could think about the following suggestions.

▶ Can you trace your back trouble to a particular activity? Gardening in a cold wind? Always carrying the shopping in the same hand? See if you can adapt the activity.
▶ What about your weight? Being overweight is an extra strain on the back.

▶ Check that your posture is good – see Chapter 4.

▶ Is your bed firm enough? Have a board put under the mattress if necessary.

▶ Try resting on the floor or other firm surface for 10 minutes at a time, twice a day. Have a firm cushion or some books under the back of the head so the neck is long. Let the small of the back sink into the floor. Lying with the knees bent, supported by cushions beneath them if necessary, is often more comfortable than with the legs straight, especially if there is discomfort in the lower back.

▶ Use this and other relaxation and visualisation techniques described in Chapter 14.

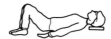

▶ Warmth – a really relaxing bath, or a hot water bottle (not scalding) in the painful place, is soothing. Gentle rubbing or massage can help too.

▶ Many people have found that treatment by a qualified osteopath brings relief.

When the pain has eased somewhat you can start to think about using the following exercises and postures. They will take your back through its normal range of movements, even if for the moment these are limited. As usual, move slowly and smoothly and listen to your body's response.

Do some stretches first to warm up and then choose one, two or three of the following sequences. Always work both sides of the body equally. And check your posture first.

If, despite investigation and treatment, you suffer from chronic pain (anywhere and for whatever reason) I can recommend an audio cassette 'Coping with Pain' produced by the Pain Relief Foundation's Pain Research Institute. Their details are in Useful Addresses at the end of this book.

STRETCHES

▶ **Side stretches** – bend to each side from the waist as far as you can comfortably go without bending forward.

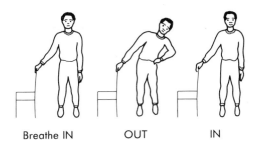

Breathe IN   OUT   IN

▶ **Four-way stretches** – remember these? The illustration shows stretches in the seated position, but remember you can do them standing up or with your feet apart if you want to.

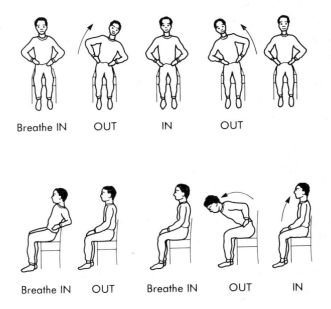

Breathe IN   OUT   IN   OUT

Breathe IN   OUT   Breathe IN   OUT   IN

HALF-MOON POSE

This is a sideways movement that can be carried out either sitting or standing.

▶ Lift one arm slowly up to the ceiling.
▶ Stretch up to the ceiling with it.
▶ Then relax your body and arm over to one side, trying not to lean forward at the same time.
▶ Come back up to the sitting or standing position and slowly drop the arm down to the side again.
▶ Repeat on the other side.

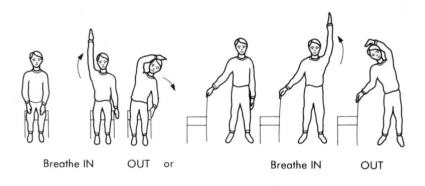

Breathe IN   OUT   or   Breathe IN   OUT

FORWARD AND BACKWARD BENDS

It is important that any forward bend is always counter-balanced with a backward stretch – this means your body is not pulled only in the one direction.

▶ To do a forward bend, sit up tall with your hands resting on your thighs. Imagine that there is a stick down the back of your jumper so you can't round your back. As you fold forward, breathe out, drawing the tummy in, keeping the back straight and the chin tucked in. Slowly straighten up into a sitting position as you breathe in, keeping the back straight and your chin in.

▶ Follow with a backward stretch. Move a little towards the front of your chair. Reach behind to hold the chair if possible. Breathe in as you arch your back, pushing the chest forward and up. Remember to keep the head straight – don't lift the chin. As you breathe out, slowly return to an upright sitting position.

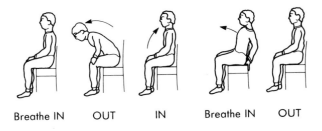

Breathe IN   OUT   IN   Breathe IN   OUT

Using two chairs

▶ Put two chairs together so that your legs are straight out in front of you – or sit on the floor if you can get down there.

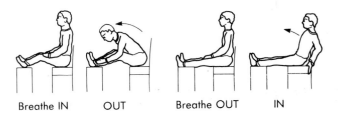

Breathe IN   OUT   Breathe OUT   IN

▶ Try some stretches, first towards the toes, then diagonally towards one foot, then the other.

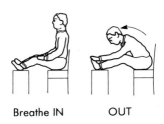

Breathe IN   OUT

TWIST AND RAG DOLL

Twist

▶ Cross your right leg over the left leg.
▶ Sit up and feel tall.
▶ Twist round and look over your right shoulder.
▶ Hold this position for a few moments, but *don't* hold your breath.
▶ Come round to the front and slowly uncross your legs.
▶ Repeat on the other side.

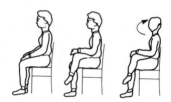

Rag doll

The twist is quite a tough movement and should be followed by a relaxing flop forward, just like a rag doll flopping forwards. Breathe out and say 'Ha!' as you flop forwards. Once you feel rested come back up slowly into the sitting position, uncurling from the base of the spine.

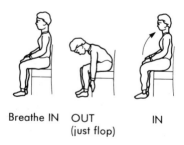

Breathe IN   OUT   IN
(just flop)

CAT

The conventional cat position is a floor exercise, and can be found on page 100. The following is an alternative that can be done standing up.

▶ Stand up straight, with your hands resting at waist level – perhaps on a chair-back.
▶ Hollow the back, trying to push your bottom up to the ceiling.
▶ Then pull in your tummy and tuck your tail under.
▶ Relax and stand up straight again.

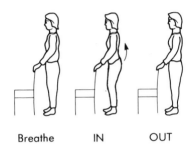

Breathe   IN   OUT

Cat variation

This is a slightly stronger variation, again standing with the hands resting on a table or chair-back at about waist level.

▶ Breathing out, lift the knee up towards the face.
▶ Breathing in, lower the leg and then raise it up behind you. Be careful not to tip forwards.
▶ Return to the standing position.
▶ Repeat three times.

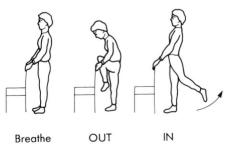

Breathe   OUT   IN

HULA HOOP

Remember the hula hoop craze in the 1960s? In this movement you should try to swivel your hips as if you were spinning an imaginary hoop round on them, first one way, then the other.

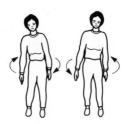

OTHER EXERCISES

You will find that many of the exercises and postures described under different headings will also help the spine, and there are more that work specifically on the back in the chapter on floor postures (Chapter 13). If you can't get down on to the floor you'll find that many of them can be done on your bed.

CHAPTER 10

HIPS AND LEGS

Legs, hips and back are inextricably linked. This is obvious if you suffer with sciatica. The pain runs down the leg, even though the cause is in the low back area where the sciatic nerve is being pinched. Strengthening the back can therefore benefit the legs, and vice versa.

HIPS

'Ladies keep their knees together.' This parental advice might have been marvellous for modesty's sake, but it didn't do much for the hip joints. In countries where squatting and sitting cross-legged are the normal thing, arthritis of the hips is practically unknown. Our 'civilised' habits and chairs have a lot to answer for! I'm not suggesting that we should take to mixing the pastry from a squatting position on the kitchen floor, or burning the three-piece suite and inviting visitors to join us on our cushions on the carpet. There are less extreme ways of making sure that we take our hip joints through the full range of their natural movement – which means prising those knees apart and opening the hips out.

Perhaps this decorous advice was given to you as a girl (gents, it seems, could sit as they pleased) and has been rigidly applied – though maybe quite unconsciously – ever since. It's hard to break such habits, but if you recognise it as one of yours see if you can learn to part the knees just enough to reduce the accompanying tension in the thighs, hips and lower trunk and yet still preserve modesty in public. When alone throw inhibition to the wind and really let go. Better still, invest in a pair of fashionable trousers and enjoy the best of both worlds.

Regularly moving the hips in the ways suggested here should not only strengthen the attached muscles and ligaments but also squeeze lubricating fluid (known as synovial fluid) round the hip joint, literally oiling it. All this can help to keep the hips strong, supple and nourished. Hopefully it will be an aid to keeping arthritis at bay, too.

If you already suffer with a stiff, painful or arthritic hip, try the movements extra slowly and carefully. It may be better to do the exercises seated rather than standing with your full weight on the uncomfortable hip. If things improve you may graduate to standing hip exercises. Do *not* work the joint while it is very painful or inflamed.

If you have had a hip replacement operation these movements can still be used, bearing in mind the usual precautions (though strong sitting twists will not be recommended). I have taught many students with one or two plastic hip joints and they have had no special problems; in fact they are usually delighted to find such freedom of movement again. If you are going in for such an operation or have recently had one, ask your doctor, specialist or physiotherapist for advice or suggestions regarding future exercise.

It is worth bearing in mind that hips are affected by posture and weight. So if you have a habit of standing or sitting with all your weight going through one hip, try to distribute it more evenly through both hips, legs and feet. We often cause an imbalance in our bodies by using one side more than the other; this applies to hips, legs and feet, in just the same way as being right- or left-handed. And again, if you are overweight this will place an extra strain on your hip joints.

KNEES

As many footballers know, knee problems can be very obstinate to treat. If you have a painful knee which is made worse by standing for any amount of time it may be better not to risk aggravating it by performing movements that make the knee take the full body weight. This may exclude standing balances such as the stork (see page 74) and even the leg raising used in the basic programme (see page 139) – even the kneeling postures, such as the cat, may need to be omitted or tried very tentatively. However there are still exercises which can benefit the knees and can be done seated. A good one is the heel-toe routine, which tones up muscles around the knee and leg without causing any strain.

Gentle massage to the knee can be helpful, provided the joint isn't red and inflamed. I know of knee sufferers (including a young rugby player) who recommend the following home treatment. Warm a little olive, castor or vegetable oil by standing a small dish of it in hot water; then rub the oil into and around the knee. This treatment can be used on other joints too – my daughter found it comforting when she suffered a 'frozen' shoulder, but only after the initial very painful stage had died down a bit.

Oil is recommended in another way for the general treatment of rheumatism. This is an old folk-remedy. A little cod-liver oil is taken morning and evening, swished up in a little fresh orange juice or milk if you can't bear it neat (it will still taste pretty horrible). Use the amount recommended on the bottle. At least it can do you no harm and I know many people who swear by this remedy, but they do say that it may be weeks, or even months, before you start to feel the benefit. Don't expect miracles overnight.

VARICOSE VEINS

Many people have varicose veins to some degree. The problem is that blood in the lower half of the body has to work continuously against gravity in order to return to the heart. This can weaken the valves in the veins (these stop the blood flowing backwards), which then don't work so efficiently. The result can be distended, throbbing veins in the legs and, when they occur in the back passage, haemorrhoids (piles).

Walking and gentle exercise is beneficial if you suffer from varicose veins. The muscle movements involved in walking stimulate the circulation and encourage the flow of blood back to the heart. In contrast, standing or sitting still for a long time will aggravate vein trouble, as will anything that hinders the circulation – sitting with the legs crossed, for example, or tight garters or elastic.

Whenever possible sit with the legs raised, perhaps on a stool.

Sometimes it helps to have the end of your bed raised on blocks. Or trying lying on the settee with your feet up on one of the arms of the settee. If you can get down on the floor, rest for a while with legs up against a wall, or on a chair. Even if you don't have varicose veins, it does us all good literally to put our feet up for a while.

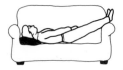 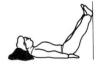 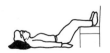

EXERCISES FOR LEGS

▶ Start with a general warm-up.
▶ Check your posture, whether you are standing or seated. Feel your weight going evenly through both hips and feet.
▶ Choose one, two or three of the following sequences, according to how you feel.

Slow-motion walk
Standing or sitting, change your weight from hip to hip. If you are standing you should be bending first one knee and then the other, as if walking on the spot in slow motion. If you are seated you will be rocking slightly from side to side. Finish with your weight evenly balanced again.

Leg swinging from the hip

▶ Standing, swing your leg loosely back and forth from the hip.
▶ Keep your back straight.
▶ Repeat on the other side.

Leg raising

▶ Check your posture – are you standing up tall?
▶ Then lift and lower each leg in turn, first forwards, then to the side and then to the back, keeping the leg straight.
▶ Hold on to a chair for support if necessary. If you do this in a seated position, omit the sideways leg raise as it is unhelpful to the knees.

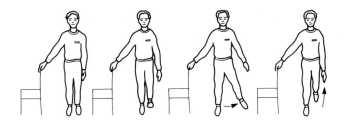

Knees up Mother Brown

Lift alternate knees as if you are climbing stairs or doing a 'knees up Mother Brown'. Again, this can be done standing or seated.

Bellows

This is a seated movement.

▶ Clasp your hands round one knee.
▶ Breathing out, lift the knee as high as it will go, pressing it towards the chest.
▶ Breathing in, lower the foot towards the floor again.
▶ Repeat three times on each leg.

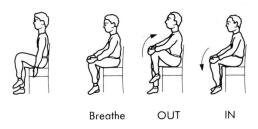

Breathe   OUT   IN

This is a variation on the usual bellows movement, which can be found in Chapter 13, the floor exercises. Alternatively, it can be done in bed.

HIP-OPENING MOVEMENTS

Leg circling

This is a standing exercise. The movement must be from the hip, not the knee or foot alone.

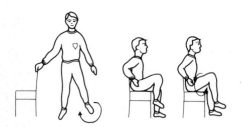

- ▶ Take all the weight on one leg.
- ▶ Start to circle your free leg from the hip.
- ▶ Start with a very small circle, then see how wide you can comfortably increase it.
- ▶ Repeat with the same leg, circling in the other direction.
- ▶ Then turn and work the other leg.

Caution: this can be quite a tiring movement. One hip has to bear all the body weight while the movement is being done. If this feels a strain try the seated version instead.

Leg circling – seated variation

- ▶ Place your hand on top of your right leg (to feel the hip joint moving), or under the knee to help it.
- ▶ Lift the right knee slightly and, keeping it bent, start to move the leg in a small circle. Can you feel the movement in your hip?
- ▶ Increase the size of the circle as desired.
- ▶ Circle in the other direction.
- ▶ Now work the other leg in the same way.

VARIATIONS OF CLASSIC YOGA BALANCING POSTURES

Stork

This is a standing-only posture that opens out the hips.

- ▶ Stand tall, with one hand on a chair-back.
- ▶ Rest your gaze on a spot ahead of you on the floor (this helps your balance).

- ▶ Feel your right leg growing strong and firm.
- ▶ Lift your left leg, turn the knee outwards, placing the sole of your foot on the inside of your right leg – ankle, calf or higher – wherever it comfortably reaches.
- ▶ Keeping straight, encourage your left hip to open out; gentle pressure with your hand will help.
- ▶ Hold the position steady for a few moments.
- ▶ Lower your leg to the ground.
- ▶ Shake both legs in turn.
- ▶ Turn and repeat with the other leg.

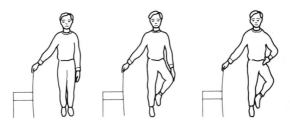

The Dancer
This is a balance that stretches the front of the thigh.

- ▶ Stand tall, with your eyes down. Picture your right leg growing firm.
- ▶ Bend your left leg. Reach behind you to hold your foot or ankle.
- ▶ Without struggling try to bring your left knee level with your right knee (pulling on the foot).
- ▶ Hold this posture for a few moments.
- ▶ Lower your leg to the floor.
- ▶ Shake both legs.

Repeat on the other side.

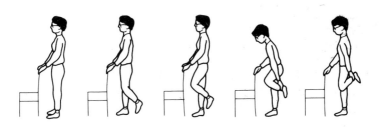

SQUATS

▶ Standing, rise up on your toes.
▶ Bend your knees (keeping your back straight).
▶ Slowly straighten your legs, rising on your toes again.
▶ Return to the standing position.
▶ Repeat three or more times, the slower the better.

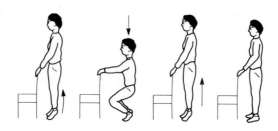

Squatting keeping your heels on the floor

Because your heels are flat on the floor, this is much harder than the previous squat. However, if you wish, you can cheat and place a book or rolled cloth under your heels.

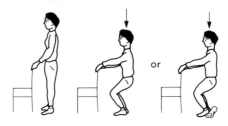

HEEL-TOE MOVEMENTS

▶ Straighten one leg at the knee.
▶ Point the toes hard away from you.
▶ Bring the toes up, push into the heel.

Repeat several times, and then repeat with the other foot.

   As an alternative you can carry out the movement with your knee bent. If you want to move your leg more, try the following variation:

▶ Straighten the leg.
▶ Push the heel away from you and bring your toes up to the ceiling.
▶ Bend your knee, bringing your foot close to the chair, and point the toes.

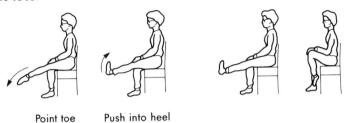

Point toe   Push into heel

This can be repeated several times, perhaps to music.

FEET

Few of us have perfect feet, and though it may be too late to change them into things of breathtaking beauty it is never too late to pay them some extra attention and make them more comfortable. Relaxing with the feet up as already described is to be recommended. Also, have a good look at your feet and what you do with them. Do you shove the poor things into narrow socks or stockings, then straight into your shoes? Is your attitude 'Let's get these unlovely things out of sight, out of mind'? The pity is that often they will *not* stay out of mind. They will protest and pinch until you have to release or rub them. We should try loving them a little instead. Find socks, stockings or tights that leave your toes free to wriggle inside them. It's no good choosing the right width shoe if your toes are already bunched up inside your hosiery. Before putting your foot into the shoe pull the stockings widthways at the toes, so they're nice and free. Then slowly slide your foot into its shoe so that your socks or stockings don't bind your feet. It may save a bit of darning too. All this may seem rather fussy, but takes very little time.

Surprising things may affect our feet – eyesight for example. I've noticed that people whose sight is poor often have stiff ankles. This may be because they become used to feeling their way with their feet and develop a shuffle, so the feet aren't used in the natural 'heel-toe' movement. The foot exercises, ankle rotation, etc., on the next page or two may help to keep them supple, as will the leg exercises described previously.

The hips affect feet, and vice versa. Check that you keep your feet parallel, especially when doing the exercises. The chapter on posture (Chapter 4) goes into this in more detail.

Tension is often obvious in feet – twitching toes, toes poking up to the ceiling or scrunched up as if to cling to the floor. These sorts of habits can all cause tiredness and aches and pains. Learning to relax your feet benefits the whole of your body. When practising relaxation we often start with the feet – as you will see later.

Meanwhile here are a few foot exercises which might help yours feel (and maybe even look) lovely.

Feet and toes

▶ If you can reach, rub all over your feet.
▶ Gently pull and separate each toe.
▶ Screw the toes under your foot, as if to pick up a pencil, then relax them.

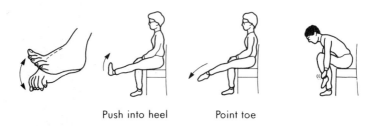

Push into heel   Point toe

▶ Pull the toes towards your shin, pushing into the heel, then point the toes away from you, then relax. Repeat several times on one foot, then repeat on the other foot.
▶ Take hold of one ankle with both hands then, keeping the foot limp, shake it. Work both feet equally.

Many postures and exercises – squats for example – will also benefit and work on your feet, particularly if they are done barefoot, without shoes and stockings.

Foot massage with no hands

This can be done either sitting or standing. Get a bottle, a tennis ball or a rolling pin, and roll it backwards and forwards beneath each foot. This is a very good way to massage your feet if you can't reach them with your hands.

CHAPTER 11

THE ABDOMEN AND PELVIC FLOOR

THE ABDOMEN

An often expressed desire by people taking up some form of exercise is 'to get my tummy down'. Unfortunately there is no magic formula. The only way to lose weight in any part of the body is by cutting down on the intake – dieting – and stepping up the output – taking more exercise. Don't be too downhearted though. Gentle consistent exercise can tone up those abdominal muscles and give you fitter flab. Improved posture will help too. It's worth noting that someone with a rotund tummy can actually have strong effective muscles under that layer of fat, while some one else with a flat stomach can still have a weak set of muscles there. A particularly chubby yoga teacher that I know does very impressive leg-raises and sit-ups (from a lying position), which require very strong abdominal muscles. I wouldn't advocate these movements for the older age group or for those who have back problems, but I will describe some exercises we can all use safely and effectively – even from a wheelchair or bed.

To achieve your target of firmer abdominal muscles, these exercises must be practised regularly – once or twice a day at least, but not on a full stomach. Unlike sit-ups, etc., they can be done anywhere, anytime – in the queue at the supermarket or at the bus stop – without causing comment. The same applies to the pelvic floor exercises.

If you are slim or unworried by a few spare tyres, is it worth bothering? Yes, definitely! Tummy muscles aren't just there for outward appearance, but to contain and support the organs inside.

Again, this applies to the pelvic floor (the sling of muscles between the legs). If you 'let it all hang out', allowing these muscles to go slack and lax, they cannot do their job so effectively. This is why digestion, elimination and reproductive organs are all helped by good muscle tone in this area.

Many of the exercises already described – such as the four-way stretch, the cat and the twist – will help tone up the abdominal muscles. However, to be effective, exercises should be done without a corset or even a lightweight girdle on. If you can bear to leave it off completely and encourage your own muscular corset to play its part, so much the better. Of course, if you have to wear a special support for medical reasons, that's a different matter. My students who wear surgical corsets still do the exercises as far as they are able.

Tummy-toning exercise

▶ Place your hands on the tummy, fingertips together (this is to feel the muscles working).
▶ Keep breathing normally. Start slowly pulling in the tummy towards the spine.
▶ As you do this, say aloud 'In ... in ... in.' This isn't a breathing instruction, it helps to make sure you're not holding your breath.
▶ When it's as flat as it will go, slowly release it letting the tummy soften, but not pushing it forward or inflating it like a balloon.
▶ Say 'Out ... out ... out' as you let go.

Do this three, six or as many times as you like, any time, any place, anywhere. I should add that it's not obligatory to keep the hands on your tum or to recite 'In ... in ... in ... out ... out ... out' in public places; it might cause comment, although on the other hand, it might liven the day up a bit.

THE PELVIC FLOOR

We don't usually think about the pelvic floor until it starts to let us down – literally. The embarassing result can be a 'leaky washer' or, in medical terms 'stress incontinence' (here the word 'stress' has nothing to do with anxiety or worry). A sneeze, laugh or cough means you have to cross your legs quickly or a few drops of urine leak out. It is often (mistakenly) seen as part of growing old, but can affect people of any age. It is more common in women, especially after childbirth. Often they will regard a certain amount of incontinence as something that has to be put up with.

In fact incontinence of this sort, and even of more severe types, doesn't have to be borne in an embarrassed silence. Mention it to your doctor so it can be investigated. It can usually be improved and often cured completely by some form of treatment. The medical profession can use a variety or combination of treatments for patients of either sex, the main ones being special exercises (on the lines of those to be described shortly), tablets (if the trouble is due to infection), appropriate treatment if it's due to sugar in the urine, and repair surgery. In men frequent visits to the toilet may be due to enlargement of the prostate gland, and medical advice will need to be taken. At the very least, if the problem is severe, professionals can help you choose aids and equipment designed to help and usually supplied by the health service.

When I first mention stress incontinence to exercise groups, embarrassment is quickly replaced by relief as students find that they are not the only ones suffering from a leaky washer or the occasional accident. I taught elderly exercise groups all through my third pregnancy and took the opportunity regularly to include pelvic floor exercises. This wasn't entirely selfless as the same movements are recommended in the months before and after childbirth, and I wanted to make sure that I kept them up and practised what I preached. And several elderly students took note of the exercises and passed them on to the mums of their latest grandchildren.

A common cause of stress incontinence in women is weakness or damage to the pelvic floor muscles which support the bladder and its outlet. During pregnancy and labour these muscles can be overstretched and damaged. Other causes are chronic constipation or persistent coughing. Doctors and specialists are quite likely to recommend pelvic floor exercises and provided these are practised conscientiously many patients have discovered that they can eliminate stress incontinence completely, sometimes doing away with the necessity for a repair operation.

Exercises to strengthen the pelvic floor

▶ This can be done sitting, standing or lying down. To identify the back half of the pelvic floor, tighten the ring of muscle around the anus (back passage). Imagine you are trying to control a bowel movement. Try not to tense the tummy, legs or buttocks while you do this.

▶ To become aware of the muscles at the front of the pelvic floor, as you pass water attempt to stop the flow in midstream (not always easy, but persevere). Try this once or twice a week.

▶ Having located these two sets of muscles, the object is to tense and relax them frequently. The idea is to work from back to front, slowly tightening the muscles and then releasing them. However this is really very hard to do, so don't worry if you can't separate back from front, but work on pulling up the whole of the undercarriage.

It's good to learn to work the pelvic floor separately from the tummy and buttock muscles, which will often want to get in on the act. You can do this by doing the following:

▶ Slowly tense the abdominal muscles only, pulling them towards the spine (as in the abdominal exercise). Then slowly release them.

▶ Tense the buttock muscles only, clenching them tightly together. Then slowly release them.

▶ Gradually tighten up the pelvic floor only, pulling up the whole area between the legs. Slowly release.

The drawbridge

This exercise we do during group exercise classes, but it is not done on a full bladder.

▶ Sit comfortably, straight but relaxed.

▶ Close or lower the eyes so you can really tune in and get the messages through to this part of the body.

▶ Let the breath flow easily – don't hold it at all.

▶ Think of your pelvic floor as a drawbridge.

▶ Slowly start to raise the drawbridge. Up . . . up . . . up . . . up.

▶ Hold it up, closed tightly (but don't hold your breath).

▶ Slowly and with control start to lower the drawbridge smoothly again.
▶ Repeat this three or more times.

When you can manage this with good control, try the following refinement. Think of raising and lowering your drawbridge in three stages. So . . .

▶ Start pulling it up, get one-third of the way, then stop.
▶ Hold it.
▶ Pull up another third, stop and hold it.
▶ Pull up the last third, so the door is completely shut.
▶ Hold it.
▶ Then slowly let the drawbridge down, third by third, pausing for one or two breaths at each stop.

At the end of exercising finish with the pelvic floor very slightly lifted, not slack.

As with any exercise, the key to success is perseverance. Like the abdominal movements, pelvic-floor tightening and releasing can be done anywhere, unbeknownst to anyone but you. You could try to do it four times every hour, or just whenever you think of it during the day. Do it every time you wash your hands after going to the loo.

Practising regularly like this, you may notice an improvement within a few weeks. If the stress incontinence is more severe it may take several months, but most students agree it is worth a try.

Incidentally, if it's of interest, such exercises are reputed to improve your love-life, too.

Some practical tips
Other things you can do to help yourself if you suffer from a tendency to incontinence include the following:

▶ As has already been suggested, consult your doctor to find the possible cause and treatment.
▶ Give yourself enough time to get to the toilet. Don't wait until you're 'desprit'. Regular toilet patterns help.
▶ If your toilet seat is awkwardly low, see about getting a gadget that makes it higher. A bar fitted for you to grab will help you up. Your doctor, health visitor or community nurse can see to these things.

▶ Think about clothing if you find it difficult to manage. Elasticated waistbands are easier to manage than buttons or zips, and Velcro flies are useful too.

▶ If you take water pills (diuretics), allow for the fact that they can cause a big increase in water passed, usually in the hour after taking them. Sleeping pills may override your natural tendency to wake up in the night when there is a need to pass water.

▶ If you find it a struggle to get to the toilet during the night, consider using a commode. They needn't be unsightly, there are many designed to look like ordinary chairs. Some people install a caravan flushing toilet, with the entry by their bed.

▶ Don't restrict the amount you drink, thinking it will help. The urine will only be more concentrated, and can actually aggravate a tendency to incontinence. If it's night-time that's the problem have your drink earlier rather than within the few hours before bed.

Over the last few chapters we've worked our way through the body, quite literally from top to bottom. In the next chapter you will find some other suggested movements which – while not yoga – will add a bit of variety to your practice. Following this, by way of a contrast there are some classic yoga floor postures which you may like to try now that you have a good grounding in the right approach.

CHAPTER 12

KEEPING EXERCISE FUN

I often think that planning an exercise routine, whether for myself or for older people or conventional yoga class, is rather like working out a menu. After a while we can fall into a habit of serving up the same familiar dishes, until the family's comments take on a subtle change. Many Mums will know the feeling. 'Oh good – it's treacle tart again' gradually changes to 'Oh – it's treacle tart again' or even to 'Oh no – it's treacle tart again.' What are needed are a few surprise ingredients in the larder. Then, when a change is needed to stop the diet becoming monotonous, we can reach in and pull one out.

I find this is particularly important when working with a regular group once or even twice a week. It's so easy to get stale. It's handy to have a list of regular menus (exercise programmes) which can be used in rotation (you'll find some in Appendix 1, and also to have a few novelties up your sleeve. Ideas for the novelties in this chapter have come from other teachers and from students themselves; we're grateful to them for letting us pick their brains.

MUSICAL INSTRUMENTS

Think of any instrument and mime it. If you are working in a group, get people to call out suggestions; piano, drums, trombone, violin – the list is endless. Make the movement large and exaggerated. The tricky bit is that both sides of the body must be worked evenly. Thus violins must be changed from left shoulder to right, trombones from one hand to the other, and even trumpeters need to move one hand up and the other down their imaginary instruments. If this sounds like chaos, just imagine the noise if the instruments materialised.

HOUSEWORK

Everyday chores can be transformed into beneficial exercise if you put your mind to it and work out ways of using the body well and evenly. Hanging out washing becomes a good stretch, weeding gives an opportunity to practise squatting, and so on. Even cleaning the bath can take on a new meaning when you think of the lovely waist bend.

IMAGINARY HOUSEWORK

On the other hand, if you feel like some exercise without the work, this can be done in a similar way to the silent musical instruments.

Cleaning windows

Imagine a huge pane of glass in front of you. Sweep your hand up and down it, working from left to right, then from side to side and/or in big circles – any way you like. Perhaps you can use great S-shaped sweeps, the way the professionals do with their big 'windscreen wiper' (I just end up with S-shaped smears when I try). Of course you must then change your wiper or chamois to the other hand and repeat the pattern of movements.

Polishing

Use wide sweeping movements as you bring a fine gloss to the great table in front of you. Lean forward as you do it so your back works as well as the arms.

Stirring the pud

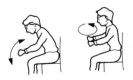

An enormous bowl of Christmas pudding mixture is sitting in your lap. You'll need two hands to grasp the wooden spoon. Stir the pud right round the edges of the bowl. Again your back will move too, in order to scrape the mixture off the sides. Change direction – from clockwise to anticlockwise. Move the hands, bottom hand to top, top to bottom, and carry on stirring.

There must be many more chores that can be adapted into exercise – wringing the clothes, rocking the baby, and so on. And sporting activities also lend themselves well – swimming, cycling, tennis, golf, archery. Just remember to use the body evenly, changing bow, bat, etc., from hand to hand.

ISOMETRICS

This sort of exercise is particularly suitable for older people. It doesn't involve any flow of movement, but muscles are made to contract by working them against resistance, such as a wall, table or other object, or by pitting the muscles against each other by simply pushing hands or feet together. As the muscles strengthen, resistance is increased. Each contraction is meant to be held for a count of four. It is very tempting to hold the breath while you do this. Don't. Just keep breathing normally. If you are specially interested in isometrics, there are books in the library and shops on the subject, but here are a few examples that we use.

Arms

▶ Place one hand on top of the other. Push one up against the downwards pressure of the other. Hold for a count of four, then reverse the hand position and repeat.

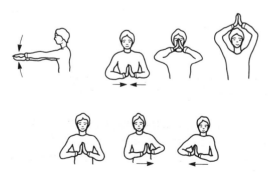

- Elbows bent, push your hands together at different heights. Hold for a count of four at each level.
- With your elbows bent, put your hands in the prayer position. Push to one side, keep up the pressure, and hold for a count of four. Push to the other side and repeat.

To release any tension created by these holds, shake out your arms and lift and drop your shoulders.

Legs

- Cross your ankles and push up with one leg, down with the other. Hold for a count of four, then change so the other leg is on top and repeat.
- Hold an object such as a wastepaper basket between your ankles. Alternatively, raise your legs slightly and place your ankles together. In either case, squeeze the ankles together or towards each other and hold for a count of four.

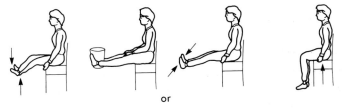

or

Other parts

Sit up straight on a dining chair, arms by your sides. Grasp the chair and try to lift your own weight. At the same time pull up with the pelvic floor. Hold for a count of four, but keep breathing.

On finishing any of these holds, shake each leg, wriggle – whatever movement your body needs to release tension.

EXERCISING IN PAIRS

This can be great fun, whether you work with your partner or with a friend. And if you are a teacher, it's an activity regular classes or groups can enjoy too, once any initial barriers are down. But remember, it might take weeks or months until the time is right, and even then, if you are running the class, allow for reticent or fearful individuals who won't want to work with anyone else. Some may join in with a little encouragement, but it's wrong to force people, however jolly your manner. For this reason pair work is only an occasional activity with most of my elderly classes; otherwise those students who really hate such things will be put off and lost to the group, and they may be the very ones who need the exercise and sociability most. Having said that, no two groups are alike, and yours may thrive on working in twos.

When you do work in a pair, be attentive to the other person – don't try and make them go further or faster than they can. It might be the end of a beautiful friendship. And don't be timid about telling your partner to slow down or go easy either. Remember the yoga principles of harmlessness and non-competition. Those who prefer to may even work solo with an invisible partner.

Pistons

▶ Sit facing your partner.
▶ Lift both arms to shoulder height, placing your palms against your partner's palms.
▶ Moving only the arms (not the back), apply a little pressure so one hand is pushed back, the other is pushing forwards.

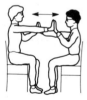 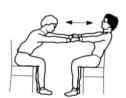

See-saw

▶ Sit opposite but slightly to the side of each other, in chairs or on the floor.
▶ Clasp hands or wrists and see-saw slowly and smoothly back and forth.
▶ If you can fit in the breathing, breathe out as you go forwards and in as you go back.

Pat-a-cake

Or 'My mother said' . . . remember this from the school playground?

▶ Clap your own hands together.
▶ You and your partner clap right hands.
▶ Clap your own hands.
▶ Clap left hands.
▶ Clap your own hands together.
▶ Clap right, then left hands.
▶ Clap your own hands together.
▶ Clap both of your partner's hands.

It helps if you chant or sing:
  Clap together – right
  Clap together – left
  Clap together – right, left
  Clap together – both.

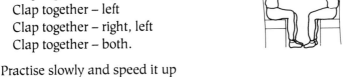

Practise slowly and speed it up
as you get it together. Don't worry if you or your partner keep going
haywire – we always do!

COUNTRY DANCING

You may be surprised to hear that you can do country dancing
from a chair. We experimented and found we could do quite a lot
of steps while sitting down. The right music helps, but fast jigs and
reels are out – find the slowest country dance music possible. I chose
a tape that I thought was quite slow enough when working the steps
out alone. First the exercise group carefully went through the steps.
Fine. Most of us had got it. Then I turned the music on. Chaos. We
all ended up in laughing exhausted heaps. Great fun, but not quite
what I'd planned!

A dance sequence can be worked out on the lines of the following
example.

Pat-a-cake-polka

Sitting in pairs or solo (clap hands with an invisible partner when
appropriate).

- ▶ Right heel to floor, right toe to floor – 4 times.
- ▶ Left heel to floor, left toe to floor – 4 times.
- ▶ Jig feet up and down as if skipping on the spot – tum te tum . . . tum te tum.
- ▶ Clap right hands together – 3 times
- ▶ Clap left hands together – 3 times
- ▶ Clap own hands together – 3 times
- ▶ Clap hands on thighs – 3 times
- ▶ Jig as before, then start again.

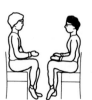

BRAIN TEASERS

I was once asked to visit a day centre for mildly confused elderly people. The plan was to go through a basic programme encouraging the patients to take their bodies through as wide a range of movement as they could manage. It was also designed to stimulate them a little and bring them out of the lethargic state into which so many seemed to have sunk.

I don't know whether it was the medication they'd been given or the close and airless room, but it was an uphill task trying to get them simply to lift an arm or shake a leg. Even enquiring about their ailments (which is usually a great conversation starter) met with a numbing silence.

In desperation I abandoned my first plan and tried a brain teaser – rubbing the tummy with one hand, patting the head with the other. (I felt there was nothing further to be lost. I looked pretty daft already, the only one doing exercises and my students dozing in a circle round me.) It worked. They sat up, paid attention and had a go. To my surprise they mastered it well. So we moved on to a more complicated one – the ear/nose trick. That went even better. After that the group were more interested in the usual exercises and attempted a few stretches and bends. After relaxation the organiser of the day centre declared that she'd never seen them so animated.

I often include this combination of mental and physical exercise in both conventional and modified yoga classes. We have a good laugh trying to do them and it's excellent practice in coordination and concentration.

Head and tum
Place your left hand on your tummy and start rubbing it in a circle. Then, while you keep that movement going, place your right hand on your head and start patting it. Keep them both going. Repeat with the right hand on the tum, the left hand patting the head. As a variation, try rubbing the head and patting the stomach instead.

Nose/ear trick
Place the right forefinger on the left nostril . . . and the left forefinger on the right ear. Got it?

Then change to your left forefinger on the right nostril . . . and your right finger on your left ear. OK?

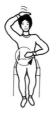

If that's easy, keep on changing, the faster the better. But mind you don't poke your eyes out!

Arm coordination
Sitting or standing, do these movements slowly and smoothly.

▶ Circle the right arm forwards a few times, then backwards. If this is too strong for you, try placing your fingertips on your shoulder and circling your elbow.
▶ Place your left palm flat on your chest. Open your arm straight so that the palm faces forwards.
▶ Then – you've guessed it – put the two movements together. Get the right arm circling first, then add the left arm opening and closing movement.

► Then circle the left arm, and open and close the right arm.

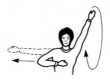

The secret of mastering this coordination exercise is to get a good rhythm going and not to move too fast.

OTHER IDEAS

Innovative students and teachers discover all sorts of activities and disciplines which can be used or adapted to older or disabled people. I know of some who incorporate T'ai chi ch'uan into such classes with great success. Television sometimes shows elderly Chinese people practising it with great dedication in their parks in the early morning. It looks like slow-motion karate. A friend who teaches T'ai chi describes it as 'a form of exercise to find stillness of mind through body movement'. Like yoga, it lends itself to adaptation for those who may have to remain seated, and if you ever have the chance to take part in such a class I can recommend it. It's certainly something I intend to take up before I draw my pension. I wonder if I'd have the guts to try it out in the local park at dawn though?

CHAPTER 13

FLOOR EXERCISES

You may like to try a few stretches and simple exercises on the floor. If you cannot get down there the first two programmes can be performed on your bed instead.

If you are working on the floor you will need a blanket or mat, one or two small cushions, and a chair.

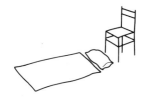

Not everybody is comfortable lying completely flat – most elderly students like to have a cushion under the head and some like to bend the knees. You should do this anyway if your back feels arched or uncomfortable.

Getting up from the floor can be the most awkward part, but don't let it put you off. At the end of the first programme there is a method which my students have found helpful.

Never rush getting up or changing from any position – lying to sitting, sitting to standing, turning onto your side or back or front. In conventional classes we all try to keep these changes slow, smooth and graceful, not just for the look of it, but to stop us going dizzy. It takes a while for blood pressure to adapt as we move from one position to another, and older people need to allow more time for this, getting up in stages and pausing when necessary. If you have someone helping you up, make sure they know this.

Each of the three following programmes lasts about 20–30 minutes. They are arranged in order so that one posture balances (or counterposes) another. The usual rules apply of finding out what is right for your body – adapt postures or don't do them if they're not right for you, if they cause discomfort or pain. Keep the movements smooth and slow. Relax and get your breath back between exercises.

PROGRAMME 1

▶ Find a **comfortable position** Place a cushion under the head or hips if necessary, or relax with the knees bent, feet hip-width apart and comfortably close to the buttocks.

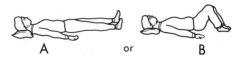

A   or   B

▶ **Relax** Feel everything becoming quiet and soft. Let the breath flow, feel the breath of relaxation (see Chapter 15) – tummy lifts as you breathe in, falls as you breathe out.
▶ **Action breaths** Deeper, more positive breathing. Raise your arms as you breathe in, lower them as you breathe out.

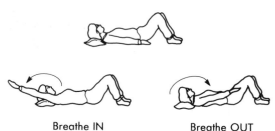

Breathe IN   Breathe OUT

▶ **Stretches (in position A)** Through the arms, then the legs, then diagonally, then right through. Keep your chin tucked in, the small of your back flat, and don't point your toes.
▶ **Bridge (in position B)** Lie on your back with your feet by your bottom and slowly raise your bottom and middle. Keep your chin tucked in. Go up and down smoothly, notch by notch. Do this three times, then rest (see page 98).
▶ **Bellows** Clasp your knees lightly on your tummy, one hand on

each knee. Gently press your knees towards your body, breathing out. Then let them relax away from your chest, breathing in. Do this six times.

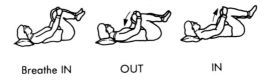

Breathe IN   OUT   IN

▶ **Relaxation**   You can do this on your back, with your knees bent if this is more comfortable, or on your side (the 'recovery position').

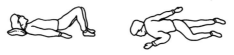

▶ **Get up slowly**   In stages – roll onto your side, push to sit up, kneel facing the chair, then use the chair to stand up slowly. Now sit on the chair for a while.

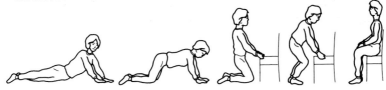

PROGRAMME 2

▶ **Relaxation**   Either lying flat on your back or with your knees bent.

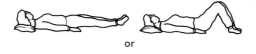

or

▶ **Stretches**   Still lying on your back, raise your arms above your head onto the floor and stretch each side, then diagonally, then right through.

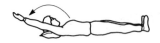

Breathe IN

▶ **Leg raising**   Bend the left knee so the foot rests on the floor by your bottom. Slowly raise the right leg (don't point your toes). Then lower the leg just as slowly, with control. Repeat on the other side. Do this three times on each side, then relax.

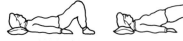

▶ **Bridge**   Lie on your back with your feet by your bottom and raise your bottom and middle, slowly peeling your back off the floor. Then lower your back and bottom smoothly and gradually down again. Do this three times.

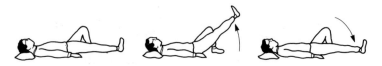

Breathe IN   Breathe OUT

▶ **Spinal rock**   Bend your knees and hug them onto your chest, then rock gently from side to side (be careful if you're doing this on your bed). Relax as the breath recovers.

 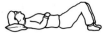 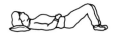

IN chest expanding   OUT tummy flattening

▶ **Breathing practice**   As you breathe in feel your ribs move upwards and outwards, and as you breathe out feel your tummy flatten out. This is the breath of action (see Chapter 15).

▶ **Deep relaxation**   In whichever is your preferred position.

PROGRAMME 3

▶ **Relaxation**   Either lying flat on your back or with your knees bent.

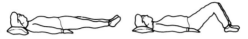

▶ **Action breaths**   Raise your arms as you breathe in and lower them as you breathe out.

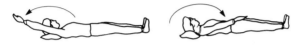

Breathe IN   Breathe OUT

▶ **Stretches**   Raise your arms above your head onto the floor and stretch each side, then diagonally, then right through.

▶ **Side leg raise**   Find your balance lying on one side, using your hands to support you, either both in front of you or one under your head and one in front of you. Slowly raise the uppermost leg, then slowly lower it. Repeat twice more.

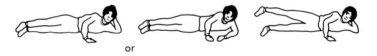

or

▶ **Cobra**   Lie face down, arms by your sides. Breathe in and slowly lift your face and shoulders from the floor. Keep your eyes to the floor, don't push your chin forward. You won't come up very far – and don't use your hands to help. Carefully lower yourself back to the floor, breathing out.

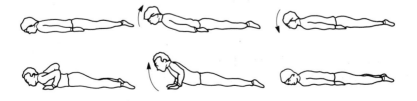

Alternatively   Lie face down with your hands beneath your shoulders. Breathing in, slowly lift your head and shoulders, then push on your hands to help. Carefully lower yourself, breathing out.

    Whichever method you use for the cobra, **relax** on your front with your head to one side and arms by your sides.

▶ **Side leg raise**   As before, but on the other side.

▶ **Relax and recover**.

▶ **Cat**   This is done on all fours, with your hands under the shoulders, knees under the hips, making a square. Breathe in, softly hollowing the back and looking up. Breathe out, pulling in the tummy, arching the back and tucking the head in. Repeat this several times, being careful not to jerk in any way.

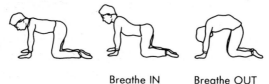

Breathe IN   Breathe OUT

▶ Rest in the **spinal rock position**, with a cushion under the head if your chin is jutting up.

▶ **Deep relaxation**   In whichever is your preferred position.

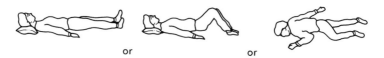

or   or

CHAPTER 14

RELAXATION

All yoga practice should start with a short period of relaxation and end with a longer one. There are often brief spells of relaxation between postures too.

Relaxation at the start of a session is to help the mind and body slow down, to let go of other preoccupations which will worry or distract the student, hindering them from reaping the full benefit. You can imagine how it is. You rush your chores in order to make time for exercise, either alone or in a group. Throwing yourself into a chair or onto your mat you think 'Thank goodness for that. Now I can do my yoga.' Then the thoughts come. 'Did I lock the door? What shall I get for dinner? Oh no, I forgot to phone so and so.' On and on it goes. How can we expect to concentrate with brains rattling on at this rate?

RELAXATION – ONE METHOD

Here's the method we use. I'll talk through it just as I would at the beginning of a class. It takes about five minutes.

Wriggle yourself comfortably into the chair (or floor).
You're sitting well – evenly and tall, neither stiff nor slumped.
Close your eyes or look down.
Take a deep breath; let out a good sigh.
Feel your body becoming heavier as you let go.
Tune in and see how you are feeling today.
If there are any tight or painful areas, talk gently to that part of the body, encouraging it to let go.
If there is a particular problem worrying you, each time that you breathe out picture the problem flowing away with the breath.
Allow your breath to flow the way it wants.

Focus on it. Feel you are watching and listening to its flow.
If your thoughts wander to other things gently bring them back to
the breath.
Don't try and control it. Let it come ... and pause ... and go ... and
pause.

At this point other suggestions can be added – details shortly.

We sit in silence for a minute or two, aware of how the body is
becoming calm and slowing down. The breath is slower and the
heartbeat too. If your blood pressure was taken it would probably
be coming down. Your thought processes have slowed too, so that
even if you haven't quite managed to take your mind off the
shopping list completely, at least you're going through it at half the
rate.
Then, as we've 20 minutes of work to do, it's time to start rousing
ourselves from this brief relaxation.
Let the breath flow more deeply, smooth and unhurried through the
nose.
Feel the energy flowing into your body, preparing it for action.
Open the eyes.
Straighten up if you've slumped a little.
Now you should feel fresh and alert, body and mind unhindered by
any tension the day might already have brought. Your mind is free
to concentrate on the task in hand so we can start – with action
breaths, stretches and warm-ups.

OTHER SUGGESTIONS

Here are some other suggestions that can be added once the
breath has settled and we are sitting or lying quietly as indicated
above.

► Describing 'Your friend the breath', as in Chapter 15 on breathing.
► Or we may feel the breath of relaxation in other ways; the cool air
flowing into the nostrils, the warmer, moist air flowing out, and/or
the gentle body movements involved – the slight expansion and lift

of the chest and upper tummy as we breathe in, the gentle fall and relaxation on breathing out.

▶ Occasionally I suggest we let any negative feelings flow out with the breath and the opposite, positive feeling flow in. So we may exhale worry, inhale peace of mind; exhale pain, inhale healing; exhale anger, breathe in tranquillity.

▶ It's good sometimes to remind students – especially new ones – not to feel guilty. Taking time off to practise relaxation is not laziness. Exercising isn't self-indulgence. We should allow ourselves time for recreation in the true sense of the word. This way we will return to our daily lives fitter in body and mind and with more energy to use for ourselves and others. I may add that it is an important preventative health measure.

RELAXATION BETWEEN POSTURES

When performing conventional yoga, with its standing, kneeling, sitting, inverted and floor postures, there will usually be a pause of a minute or two between groups of postures so that students can lie down on the floor and practise relaxation. This is done in much the same way as I have just described. As yoga students become used to this they usually learn to 'switch off' and relax almost instantly. Then, however brief the interval, they are able to continue with no breathlessness or tension carried over into the next exercises or postures.

The same applies whether you're practising by yourself or in a group. Heed your body. If it is tired or starting to feel strained, or if you are becoming breathless, rest for a few moments until you have recovered. Your breath is really the best guide. This applies as much when using your gentle exercise routines as it does with conventional yoga. Even though time is limited, we must pause when we need and sit quietly. Sometimes we'll talk a little about what we've just done, to give time to those who need it. More energetic movements – such as the Four-way Stretch – will be followed by an easier one, perhaps finger-presses or eye exercises. Students are always advised to rest when they need until they're ready to join in again, even if it means letting the rest of the group continue. Just sit quietly and let the breath flow. A few deep breaths or sighs first of all will help. Don't hold on to the breath. Go with it. Students of all ages find that one of the benefits of yoga is that their recovery rate becomes much quicker even after violent exercise, whether chasing a bus or marathon running.

RELAXATION TO END A YOGA OR GENTLE EXERCISE SESSION

First make sure that conditions are right, especially that you will be warm enough. We cool off quickly once we sit or lie still. Have a woolly or a blanket handy. You may stay seated in your dining chair or you may prefer an armchair. Though your posture is bound to soften as you relax, start with a good tall position, not slumped, or breathing will be hindered. You may prefer to lie on the floor (see the floor exercises in Chapter 13) or relax in bed.

If you find certain music helps you unwind, have it within reach and switch it on whenever you choose. If you are in a group it may be better to leave it until the relaxation has been talked through (background music during verbal instructions may make it difficult for people who are hard of hearing).

There is a lovely variety of ways to encourage a good relaxation. One may work better than another for you, but it's nice to experience several and (as in the postures) keep a variety in your repertoire.

In the following paragraphs I will talk you through a 10-minute relaxation I often use at the end of a basic programme. It is a good introduction to the art of relaxation. Descriptions of other techniques will follow shortly.

If you are doing this by yourself, read the instructions through, get the general idea, shut the book and off you go. It doesn't really matter if you forget little bits or do them in a different order. However, if you are in a group or class, one person can read the instructions clearly and slowly and loud enough for everybody to hear without straining. When I am conducting the relaxation I always reassure students that the list contains only suggestions; each person is free to do as they wish. Even when completely relaxed *you* are still in charge.

Try to remain aware of the suggestions and resist the temptation to fall asleep immediately. However, if you realise afterwards that you did nod off or lose track – well, it really doesn't matter at all.

TOE-TO-TOP RELAXATION

The first group of instructions are a good way with which to start any relaxation period.

Settling down

Wriggle yourself well into the chair.
Hands rest quietly in your lap.
Feet heavily on the floor or cushion.
Close eyes or look down.
Accept that there will be some level of noise, even if it's just the ticking of a clock. Let life go on around you.
Turn **within** to that quiet centre.
Sigh deeply ... and again.
Let the **breath settle** and come and go of its own accord.

Systematic tension release

So that we can tell the difference between a state of tension and relaxation we are going to work through the body, first tensing, then releasing each part in turn.

▶ Take your attention to your **feet**. Screw up the toes tightly then let them soften. Lift your feet off the floor and let them drop. They will remain still and heavy.

▶ Tighten up your **calves** then let them go soft.

▶ Pull your **knees** tightly together, release them and allow them to stay parted a little.

▶ Tense up the big muscles of the **thighs**. Feel them pushing against the chair. Now let them go.

▶ Pull your **buttocks** together. Now release and let your bottom sink into the seat of the chair.
▶ Tighten everything between the legs, pulling up your **under-carriage**. Tight ... tighter ... now slowly let it go.
▶ Pull your **tummy** in towards the spine. Slowly release.

Now all the lower part of your body feels heavy and relaxed. Let it rest in this way while we take our attention to:

▶ **Hands** – clench them into fists, then stretch out the fingers and let them relax and curl the way they want to. Lift the hands and drop them onto your lap. Let them rest where they fall.
▶ Tense your **arms** (keeping hands relaxed still). Let them go.
▶ Lift your **shoulders** a little. Now let them drop.
▶ Your **chest** feels open and free, moving gently as the breath comes and goes.
▶ Your **neck** feels comfortable, straight in line with the spine.
▶ Be aware of your **jaw**. Clench the teeth together. Feel the tension. Now release and let the teeth part.
▶ Screw up your whole **face**. Let it smooth out slowly, **cheeks** soft, **eyelids** heavy.
▶ Raise your **eyebrows** as if very surprised. Let them go. Feel there's lots of space between the brows.
▶ Let go of any tension round your **ears**.
▶ Even your **scalp** feels a little looser now.
▶ It's nice at this stage to picture relaxation climbing the **spine**. Take your attention to its base and imagine relaxation slowly rising, like mercury in a thermometer. As it climbs you can feel that part of your back letting go. Pay particular attention to the area between the shoulder blades – a place where tension often starts.

Rest in relaxation
Your whole body is now in a pleasantly relaxed state.

▶ Your **breath** comes and goes, flowing the way it wants, like waves breaking on the shore, taking away any remaining tension, bringing in relaxation.
▶ For the moment we will just enjoy this feeling of calm and quietness.
▶ As our bodies have quietened so our thoughts will have slowed

too. Don't try and make the mind a blank. Be aware of your thoughts. Don't concentrate on any one in particular. Watch them coming and going like trains through a station.

At this point we rest in silence or with a background of soft, pleasant music.

After a minute or two we move on to the next stage. If you are taking the class, don't leave it too long; if the class are sitting in hard chairs the older people may either start getting stiff and uncomfortable or gradually list too far and lose their balance. If you have this fear use a chair with arms. Getting the fidgets means you've had long enough.

Come round slowly
In many yoga classes the teacher will now say 'Om chanti chanti om', the yoga words for 'peace'.

▶ Bring your **thoughts** back to here and now.
▶ Without opening your eyes, be aware of the weight of your **body** again and its position in the chair, its place in the room.
▶ Tune in again to the **sounds** going on around us.
▶ Allow the **breath** to flow more deeply, bringing in energy ready to move again.
▶ Move the **head** slightly from side to side.
▶ Wriggle the **fingers** and **toes**.
▶ **Straighten** up if you've slumped a little.
▶ Have a really good **stretch** any way that you need. Yawn, sigh, whatever your body tells you.
▶ Open your **eyes** if you haven't done so.
▶ **Smile**.

NOTE If you have enjoyed a really deep relaxation and your body is slow or reluctant to come round count slowly from 10 to 1, knowing that number 1 represents full alertness. It may take quite a bit of practice to get the knack of relaxation. Be patient, persevere and try different methods – one may just 'click'.

Don't rush off as soon as relaxation has ended. You may feel rather slow and dreamy at first. That's good. A little later there may be a surge of energy which thorough relaxation can release.

VARIATIONS

There are many ways of talking the body into releasing tension and entering a state of relaxation. Here are some that we use.

Letting each part go in turn

This is done the same way as already described but, instead of tensing first, think your way through the body, feeling every part softening and releasing. You could work from top to toe for a change.

Talking to yourself

Say to yourself 'My right foot is heavy and warm ... My left foot is heavy and warm ...', talking through each limb in turn until 'My whole body feels relaxed and at ease.'

Picturing heat

This is useful in chilly weather. Start with your feet, picturing a gentle warmth – like a candle flame perhaps – beneath your soles, slowly spreading through the toes, ankles, lower legs, knees, thighs, etc. The glow can climb the spine too.

Count-down to relaxation

You are going to breathe in and out ten times, each breath taking you down into deeper relaxation. Count them, starting at ten and ending on one. You are then at a deep level of relaxation and can use a visualisation if you wish.

To 'come round', count the breaths up again to full alertness.

VISUALISATION

This means using the 'mind's eye' to help relaxation.

Once in a relaxed state, scenes can be brought to mind which will enhance relaxation and encourage a calm and positive state of mind. Some people refer to this practice as imagery, others as visualisation or meditation. You could even call it daydreaming. Whatever name you use, I'm sure you'll find it an enjoyable thing to do and will be able to think of your own personal experiences to draw on.

Special place

A special place can be pictured in the mind's eye. It can be real, somewhere from the past, or completely imaginary. It might be a garden, a room, the sea or countryside – anything that appeals to you and makes you feel happy and at ease. Picture the shapes and colours – the blue of the sky, the colours of the flowers, etc. Hear the sounds – birdsong, waves on the shore, the hum of insects, etc. Feel the sensations – the gentle sun on your face, a playful breeze perhaps, even the scents you would find there. Enjoy your special place with all of your senses. As you finish your relaxation let the picture fade, but remember that place and others like it are always there within you to draw on when you need.

Walk in the country

Picture the countryside in whatever season you choose. Walk down a path. Follow it through fields, drinking in all the scene (as above). Perhaps you will choose to pass through a pleasant wood or beside a stream before you return to the place from which you started.

A tree

See a bare tree, then slowly and in great detail watch it blossom. Or picture it going through each season in turn.

A warm beach

Picture yourself on a warm beach and watch the sun setting on the sea.

POSITIVE THINKING

Sometimes when you do these visualisations (especially if you are feeling low) see yourself as you wish to be – as you can be – well, happy, at ease with yourself, full of energy.

Someone you care for

If you are concerned about someone you care for picture that person not as they are (perhaps tired, ill, fearful or unhappy) but as you would like to see them – well and happy. Picture a warm glow and place your friend or loved one in it.

We have done this as a group, perhaps centring on one person in particular. It can be a comforting and healing experience for everyone. It's good to turn energy spent on worry into something more positive.

Dancing

See yourself moving freely and easily in time with the music. Dance with a chosen partner if you wish.

Healing

If some part of your body is stiff or painful, has been troubling you or isn't functioning as well as it might, focus on that part. 'Breathe into it' – picture light, colour or warmth flowing into that place and as you breathe out feel that you are breathing away the problem.

Hot-air balloon

Picture a hot-air balloon resting in a field, its large basket on the grass, the balloon deflated. Package any problems you wish to be rid of – anger, pain, tiredness. Place these negative things in the basket until it is piled high. Then watch the balloon inflate and slowly leave the ground, taking off into a clear blue sky. Watch it grow smaller and smaller until it disappears altogether, leaving you feeling unburdened and peaceful.

MORE ABOUT VISUALISATION

As well as using visualisation to enhance relaxation, it has a valuable role to play during postures and exercises too. Its use can make a surprising difference. Demonstrate this to yourself by trying the following experiment.

Turn the head slowly to look over the left shoulder, keeping the rest of the body straight. Without straining, see how far you can see behind you. Notice the furthermost object. Straighten the head once more and close the eyes. Now imagine that you have a neck like an owl's. Picture your head turning smoothly to the left until you are 'looking' down your spine. With this picture firmly in your mind open the eyes and turn the head to the left again. Before straightening up note the furthermost point or object. Any difference?

Many students find that they can see further behind them the second time. The visualisation seems to increase the neck movement but causes no strain. (This should then be repeated on the right side.)

Visualisation is a useful tool when your body is limited in its range of movement. For example, if you cannot lift a limb far (or even at all), close your eyes and picture it moving as it should. I know it sounds daft, but it does seem to help. In the same way, if you have a particular joint which is affected by stiffness, rheumatics or arthritis when you are relaxing – perhaps in bed at night – imagine it working well. Some folk I know conjure up an oil can, and grease their tricky joint. Then picture it going through its full range of movement or doing something you find difficult, whether it's playing the piano or walking upstairs. Do it smoothly and easily in your mind's eye.

Imagery can be used to back up conventional medical treatment too, picturing the pills, physiotherapy, whatever, working well and bringing about improvement.

Visualisation in fact can be put to so many uses. If you are painfully shy, imagine yourself in a situation where you have to meet people but see yourself as more confident, greeting and talking to people. (You have to give yourself a chance to practise it in real life too.)

Some people would describe these methods as 'mind over matter' but that can imply a forceful approach. The beauty of visualisation is that it is a gentle method, rather like encouraging good behaviour in a child through praise instead of punishment.

You might think that we have wandered from the original heading of this chapter. In fact it's been found that combining relaxation with visualisation at the end of a gentle exercise programme has helped so many new students really to let go that one couldn't be described without the other. A remarkable incident illustrated this the other day. Mrs Price has Parkinson's disease, which gives her hands a constant, uncontrollable tremor. About the fifth week that she attended classes I noticed that during relaxation, while we were visualising a garden scene, her hands were resting completely still in her lap. She commented on how she'd enjoyed relaxation that day, but was quite unaware that the shaking had stopped for a while. She was thrilled to realise that it had done so. This illustrates not only the remarkable and often inexplicable link between mind and body, but also that it is possible for elderly people (after a little practice) to relax deeply and effectively within a few minutes – even on a hard chair.

The way you breathe plays an important part in being able to relax as well. It is yet another of nature's tools which can improve general health, relieve stress and generally help us function better. The next chapter will show how.

CHAPTER 15

BREATH OF LIFE

If you have been following this book and practising some of the exercises, postures and relaxation you will already have laid the foundation for improved breathing. Now you might like to think about this function in more detail and try some simple breathing exercises.

You may wonder what's so special about breathing – you've been doing it for years. But few of us do it well. When we are babies our breathing follows a natural pattern, ideally suited to our needs. Unfortunately, as we grow up the stresses and strains of daily life, and even the clothes we wear, often mean that we no longer make full use of our marvellous breathing equipment. Many of us develop the habit of breathing too shallowly, too fast or too heavily.

Poor breathing can affect our health and also our state of mind. Listen to your breath now. Is it smooth, rhythmical and quiet? If so you will be feeling relaxed and calm. If it is shallow, quick and/or heavy, watch for other signs of tension – raised shoulders, clenched teeth, frown lines. Quieten the breathing and the mind will follow – tension will be released.

If you purposely make yourself breathe very fast and jerkily you will soon start to feel anxious, even panicky. *Don't* try it – just take my word for it. Fortunately it works the other way round too, so when we are feeling tense or panicky a few slow deep breaths will help us to regain a calm mind and body. Try this the next time you feel yourself getting in a state. I remember when I became cross or excited when I was little my granny would often tell me to take a deep breath and count to ten, so you see breathing advice is nothing new.

Special use of the breath can have remarkable effects on the body, especially in its ability to heal and revitalise itself. Philip Jones is an example of this – and to us all. Pneumonia as a child, plus a subsequent mining career, left him with severely damaged lungs. Inhaled coal dust had formed a tar-like deposit in the bottom of his lungs, making breathing more and more difficult; called pneumoconiosis, this disease is said to be irreversible. No longer fit and active, Philip passed his time reading widely. One day, he chanced upon a yoga book from the library and it opened a whole new world for him. He learnt correct breathing and practised intense yoga breathing exercises. The result is that Philip now lives a full and energetic life, travelling the country teaching yoga, passing on his knowledge and helping many people – particularly those with chest complaints. Philip tells me that he feels it is possible to control pneumoconiosis through yoga; its practice has expanded the capacity of his chest and lungs, perhaps bringing into use areas of the lungs which aren't generally used.

We shouldn't expect breathing exercises to bring about a miracle cure, but we can all benefit from becoming aware of the breath, learning to breathe properly and doing a few simple breathing exercises every day. And how does it help? Well, the cells of our body need oxygen to survive. Breathing *in* deeply brings in a good supply of oxygen and energy (and, according to yoga beliefs, that indefinable thing – prana – the life force). Breathing *out* well lets out the used air (and carbon dioxide), leaving your lungs ready for fresh supplies again.

In order to improve the way you breathe the following sequence of breathing exercises – the breath of relaxation and the breath of action – are the most important ones to practise.

BREATH OF RELAXATION

You can use this while lying on the floor (see Chapter 13 on floor postures), on your bed or sitting well in an upright chair.

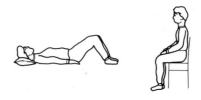

Sit or lie quietly. Become aware of the flow of your breath, let it come and go of its own accord, don't try to control or force it. No effort or noise is necessary. Your face should be smooth, shoulders loose, chest not held stiff. You should feel nicely relaxed. Only the abdomen moves – tummy rising slightly as you breathe in and falling as you breathe out. This isn't a deliberate pushing out or pulling in, but merely the result of the air inside the lungs coming and going.

You will probably find that the out breath is longer and more obvious than the in breath. That is the way it should be – the out breath is the more important and as you naturally pause after breathing out you will find that air will 'sneak' or float in again when the body needs it.

A suggested visualisation

My students have found the following suggestion useful when practising this relaxed breathing.

Think of your breath as a friend and your body as your house. Just as you wouldn't drag your friend in roughly or force him out of your house before he is ready, so it is with your friend the breath. Let him come and go as he pleases. Don't rush him – he will probably want to pause for a moment after he's entered and again after he's left.

This friend is an especially good and obliging one when you come to think of it. When he comes into your house (body) he brings a marvellous gift – life and energy to every cell – and when he leaves he takes the rubbish with him.

BREATH OF ACTION

Still in the same relaxed (but not slumped) position you are going to change to taking control of the breath, making it deeper, more positive, and encouraging the correct movement of the body. Breathe through the nose if possible, though you may need to take the first one or two breaths through the mouth.

► As you slowly and smoothly breathe in, feel the ribs move upwards and outwards, with as wide a movement as possible.
► As you breathe out gradually flatten your tummy, slowly drawing it backwards towards the spine.

▶ Take your time, but don't try to breathe so slowly or deeply that it feels a strain.

The basic idea is very simple: the body expands as you breathe in, and becomes smaller as you breathe out.

Test yourself

Here's a way to check that this is happening. Place your hands, fingertips touching, an inch or two above your navel. Use the action breaths just described.

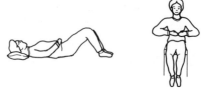

As you breathe in, deeply and smoothly, do your fingertips part a little? (Remember the movement should only be gentle – don't push the abdomen forward.) As you breathe out, smoothly and controlled, the fingertips should move together again as the abdomen flattens and the rib-cage becomes smaller.

And what if your fingertips stay together and nothing seems to be moving? Well, this gives you something to work on. Don't be discouraged if it takes a lot of practice to get it right. A lifetime's habit will take time to change.

WHEN TO USE THESE BREATHS

Practise the breath of relaxation and the breath of action until you can go from one to the other and back again. In the end it will become quite smooth and effortless. That is what we are aiming for.

Specifically, you can use the breath of action:

▶ to wake you up in the morning
▶ to prepare for action after relaxation
▶ and at the beginning and end of a gentle exercise or yoga session.

You can then go on to use these action breaths linked to arm movements, stretches and postures. The illustrations throughout the book show you where it is appropriate to breathe in and where to breathe out. Again, it may take quite some time before it all fits smoothly together – it seemed years before I could get the breathing for the cat stretch right, and I still have to think about it now. In the meantime the important thing is not to hold your breath, and *keep breathing*!

Of course you can't go around breathing deeply all day – you'd soon find all that oxygen making you light-headed. However if such breathing is practised for just a few minutes each day the lungs will gradually work better, even when you're not thinking about it, and gradually the habit of breathing in a shallow and restricted way will be lost.

SOME SIMPLE YOGA BREATHING EXERCISES

The bee breath

▶ Take a smooth, long breath in through the nose.
▶ Hum for the length of the exhalation (the out breath).
▶ Repeat twice more.

Don't try to make the out breath longer than comes naturally to you, or it will feel and sound strained. Humming has a calming effect and, I think, lifts the spirits (have you ever heard someone humming when they're miserable?). It is said to induce relaxation and sleep. It's certainly a nice way to practise extending the out breath, and many elderly students have surprised themselves by the length of their exhalations when humming.

It's lovely to do the bee breath in a group – whatever note you hum on, all the tones blend together beautifully. You don't have to be a singer; simply choose whatever note you like. And there's no need to feel self-conscious, as everybody closes their eyes and you can't tell who's humming what.

Cleansing breath

▶ Breathe in through the nose as fully as possible.
▶ Lightly clench the teeth and hiss out the breath for as long and as fully as you can without straining.
▶ Repeat twice more.

Tension-releasing breath

This exercise is done seated. It has a cleansing effect on the mind and body and is the thing to do when you are feeling angry or generally frustrated – it is certainly cheaper than throwing crockery, and kinder than kicking the cat. A great way of letting off steam.

▶ Press the palms of the hands together hard. Feel the physical tension flowing through your hands, arms, shoulders and chest. This is symbolic of the emotional tension that can build up in us.
▶ Start breathing in, deep and long, and at the same time push the hands (heels of the hands still together) up towards the ceiling. Picture whatever feeling you wish to be rid of resting in your hands and being pushed up . . . up . . . away from you, ready to be released.

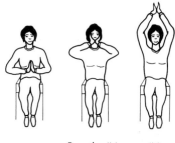

Breathe IN   IN

▶ Breathe out, through the mouth this time, hissing noisily through the teeth, like a steam train at the end of its journey. A genteel little 'sssss' just will *not* do.
▶ At the same time let the arms fall limp and heavy, and let your trunk go too as you relax, releasing that negative feeling you've been holding on to.
▶ Straighten up slowly with your chin tucked in.

► Repeat twice more.

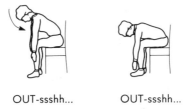

OUT-ssshh...   OUT-ssshh...

Students of all ages have said how effective they have found this exercise.

Using the breath as a concentration exercise
This is described in the next chapter on page 127.

IMPROVING YOUR BREATHING

As well as practising breathing exercises, there are other things you can do to encourage better breathing in everyday life and to get the most out of your gentle exercise and breathing sessions.

► Breathe through your **nose**, unless this is impossible for you. Your nose is a wonderful cleansing and air-conditioning system. That's what it's there for.
► Improve your **posture**. Check it specially before breathing practice. There's never any excuse to slouch! Keeping your spine long (not stiff) and your chest open gives your lungs room to work properly. Any chest complaint will be aggravated by rounded shoulders and a caved-in chest.
► **Don't smoke.** Sorry smokers, you knew I was going to say that. We can't get away from the fact that smoking – whether cigarettes, cigars or a pipe – plays havoc with just about every part of the body but especially the lungs. Give up, or at the very least cut down *now*. It's never too late, and many students find that the combination of physical exercise, breathing and relaxation helps them give up and lessens the craving. If you need help to give up, your GP may be able to advise you.

▶ Avoid being a **passive smoker.** This means trying to keep out of other people's smoky atmosphere. This can be tricky. My mother (a non-smoker) had a terrible smoker's cough in the morning until Dad agreed not to light up his pipe in the bedroom.

▶ It's good to do some deeper breathing, such as the breath of action, in the **fresh air,** but *not* in the icy blast from a window, nor in bitter or foggy conditions outside.

▶ **Don't strain.** If you feel breathless or need to sneak in extra breaths you're trying too hard.

▶ See how much **suits you.** Don't practise deep breathing for more than a few minutes at a time. Feeling light-headed means you're overdoing the oxygen intake.

▶ **Be patient.** Breathing's a bit like walking – if you think about it in detail you're apt to fall over. If you find it hard to practise as an isolated activity, concentrate on doing the physical exercises in which good chest expansion and body movements tie in with a breathing pattern; for example swimming and its variations (page 56), **swimming in space** (page 147), cow head (page 57), the cat (page 100) and the bellows (page 73 or 96).

▶ All the breathing suggestions in this book are safe for a beginner, elderly or handicapped person. If you feel you would then like to go on to more **advanced breathing** techniques it would be best to find a yoga teacher to guide you.

▶ And an important footnote. **Laugh** as often as you can – it's the best breathing and relaxation exercise in the world!

IF YOU HAVE A CHEST COMPLAINT

People with asthma, emphysema, bronchitis and other chest conditions can benefit tremendously from practising gentle exercise, relaxation and breathing exercises. Of course, you should take note of the advice given above for improving your breathing, but in addition here are some further points.

You should work particularly on the breath of relaxation (page

114). Once you have mastered this – and it may take some time – you can then concentrate on the breath of action (page 115). Then work on action breaths (page 42), mountain breaths (page 42) and other arm movements linked to the breath. The cleansing (hissing) breath should be helpful too (page 118). Most importantly, you should **never** try to do exercises while the chest is in spasm.

If you suffer from asthma or other chest conditions you may find that you can't lie completely flat or on your tummy. This is where the seated exercises come into their own. But suppose your body is willing and able to get down on the floor, if only to try the relaxation positions? Well, you will probably then be more comfortable there with your back well propped up with cushions.

If your chest condition doesn't hinder you from using some of the simple floor postures described in this book, I can specially recommend the bridge (page 98). Later you could try the cobra (page 100).

Other things that can be helpful include avoiding being overweight. And don't get overtired – have some early nights if you feel low.

VISUALISE HEALTH

A nd all of us can benefit from using visualisation to aid breathing.

▶ As you breathe in picture energy (prana) bringing relief, health, strength, warmth and good posture.
▶ As you breathe out breathe away infection, tension, shallow breathing, mouth breathing and germs.
▶ Picture your lungs glowing with **health!**

CHAPTER 16

Exercising your mind

In Chapter 1 'Use it – don't lose it' I described how experts now believe that much of the absent-mindedness of which adults complain is not due to the brain cells dying, as many people believe. So, unless you are suffering from an actual disease which affects the brain – and old age *isn't* a disease – there is still hope (or no excuse, whichever way you like to look at it). Much forgetfulness in life is due to lack of concentration, on becoming distracted by all the other things our mind is rattling on about. My daughter is so involved with her French studies she forgets to phone her friend. I'm so busy stacking the shopping away before my visitor arrives a brand new pair of tights ends up in the freezer.

Concentration, like all other skills, improves with practice. I've found that older people seem able to apply themselves better to concentrating during both physical and mental exercises. Perhaps this is because they grew up in an era that moved at a slower rate, or perhaps it's because their lives are no longer lived at such a hectic pace. Just to sit still and focus on one thing alone seems much more difficult for younger generations.

Concentration and meditation go hand in hand, though I can't tell you where one ends and the other starts. The following definition is one I like.

► **Concentration** is when you focus your attention on an object but at the same time you are aware of other distractions – noises, other thoughts and so on; in spite of them, you keep taking the mind back to its chosen focus.

► **Meditation** is when you become aware only of the object of the concentration, so that you are no longer aware of other distractions.

I call the mental exercises I am going to describe concentration, and if they lead on to what you would describe as meditation, that's fine.

And there's nothing weird about concentration/meditation. You've probably been doing it for years. (I'm very aware that I'm often 'teaching granny to suck eggs'.) Like the old man who spends hours sitting tranquilly in his chair. 'Sometimes I sits and thinks', he explains, 'and sometimes I just sits.' And then there's the poem 'Leisure' by William Henry Davies:

> What is this life if, full of care,
> We have no time to stand and stare? . . .
> No time to stand beneath the boughs
> And stare as long as sheep or cows.

Normally our minds are very restless, with thoughts flying all over the place, rarely settling for long. Becoming used to periods of quiet concentration will eventually help the mind to concentrate better in everyday life, whatever the task in hand.

POSSIBLE BENEFITS

And there are other benefits too. Practising concentration/ meditation in the correct (relaxed) way helps physically too, often producing changes that can actually be measured. During a meditative state, blood pressure can become lower and brainwave patterns change from a typical waking pattern to nearer the sleeping state. So the body lets go and relaxes more deeply. This is why more and more doctors are recommending meditation classes for patients with high blood pressure, migraine, asthma, anxiety and other stress-related conditions. And why some practise what they preach and set aside time to do it themselves.

The physical changes that take place may be one reason why so many people say they feel refreshed and their batteries recharged afterwards. As one older student, Miss Robinson, put it, she could 'climb mountains'. Sometimes we become so preoccupied with some worry or other that it is on our minds all the time. Totally occupying the mind with something else is a great relief. Afterwards things can seem in better proportion. This is an experience common among all ages.

PREPARING FOR RELAXED CONCENTRATION

So, a period of relaxed concentration refreshes mind, body and spirit. However, to concentrate in the right way needs a little preparation. The body must be comfortable and the breath flowing easily. Some gentle exercise or a few stretches beforehand will help. If you are using a gentle exercise or yoga programme, concentration fits nicely in the slot before the final relaxation period – in fact it can merge into it.

You can concentrate by yourself or in a group. Ideally your surroundings should be quiet, though there may always be some distractions (even if it's just the ticking of a clock) and these must be accepted. You could take the phone off the hook for five minutes though. It's better not to lie down to concentrate – it's too easy just to doze off. Sit in a comfortable chair with your back straight, but not stiff, so you feel balanced and your breathing isn't hindered.

Let go of any tension. And don't forget to relax your face. You don't need to frown or tense up while concentrating; 'calm looking' is what you're aiming for. You could sigh deeply once or twice and then let the breath quieten and settle. This is the breath of relaxation, described in Chapter 15 on breathing. You are now ready to enjoy a period of concentration on an object of your own choice. It can be an everyday thing such as an apple.

SOME CONCENTRATION EXERCISES

An apple
For our first concentration exercise we'll start by noticing how, without the gentle discipline of concentration, our thoughts usually tend to run away by themselves. It's a word association game.

Think of an apple, then say the first word that comes into your head associated with an apple, then a word associated with that word, and so on. It might go something like this:

Apple→Tree→Leaf→Flower→Roses→Anniversary→Aunt Betty→Mauve hair

See how far your thoughts have strayed already.
Now we'll practise concentration.

▶ Look at your apple.
▶ Really look.
▶ See the colours, the light and shade.
▶ Feel the shape, the skin texture.
▶ Smell the apple. Savour its fruity scent.
▶ Close your eyes softly.
▶ Imagine the taste.
▶ If you cut it in half, what would it look like inside?
▶ Picture the flesh, the core, the pips.
▶ Shake it by your ear – sometimes you can hear the pips rattle.
▶ Use all your senses to get to know your particular apple.
▶ Let your thoughts return to it again and again, gently resisting the temptation to let your thoughts wander away as they did before.

You are now practising concentration. How long you take is up to you – five or ten minutes perhaps. Then, leaving the eyes closed, take your focus from the apple and enjoy a few moments relaxing and feeling at peace.

Come round slowly, stirring and stretching and taking a few deeper breaths – just as you would when finishing an ordinary relaxation.

If your body is slow or reluctant to come round count slowly from 10 to 1, knowing that number 1 represents full alertness.

A flower

▶ Hold the flower loosely in your hand.
▶ Absorb its shape, the way the petals are arranged.
▶ Can you see its centre (as in a daisy)?
▶ Notice the colours and the way they blend into one another.
▶ Feel the textures of the different parts – the stem, the petals, a leaf perhaps.

▶ Does it have a scent?

▶ Look at your flower in its completeness. Perhaps it wouldn't be considered a perfect specimen, but its very flaws can make it more individual, more interesting.

▶ Imagine you are going to paint it and capture its likeness on paper. Close your eyes and (keeping your face soft) see your flower in your mind's eye.

▶ If you lose the image – open your eyes and look again.

▶ Remember the feel of the different parts, the scent too.

▶ You may like to take your picture further. Imagine how your flower would look if you were as small as an insect. Feel a petal supporting you.

▶ Wander among the petals and stamens, seeing the colours close and vivid.

▶ Enjoy it with all of your senses.

▶ Then picture the flower as it is, resting in your hand, once more.

▶ Slowly let the picture fade.

▶ Savour the pleasant sensation it leaves in your mind

▶ Pause in this relaxed state as long as you like.

▶ Come round slowly.

A candle flame

A candle flame is a traditional concentration exercise. I think it's not unlike the way people sit and gaze into the fire on a cold winter's night. Central heating has its benefits, but also at least one disadvantage!

If you wear glasses it's probably best to remove them first, unless it makes vision strained or impossible. It won't hurt your eyes, though if you have a particular problem such as extreme light sensitivity or double vision this would not be a suitable exercise for you as it might be a strain. Blink whenever you need to, but don't be surprised if your eyes water a bit – think of it as a cleansing.

Here's what you do. Sit in a comfortable but not slumped position, as before. Have in front of you (ideally an arm's length away and at eye level) a lighted candle.

▶ Relax and let your breathing settle.

▶ Let your gaze rest on the candle flame.

▶ Observe its shape, colours, warmth and the glow, the aura around it. Take your time.

▶ Softly close your eyes and picture the flame and everything you saw. This will be helped by the image of the flame being imprinted beneath the eyelids.

▶ Observe the image and the way it changes. It may be all sorts of colours and the size may vary – it's different for everybody.

▶ Try, without straining, to keep the flame in the centre of your field of vision – it will want to dart off in all directions.

▶ If it disappears or becomes so small it fades away, open your eyes and look at the flame again for a while.

▶ When you have concentrated as long as you wish let the image and the control go. Just rest quietly.

Come round slowly as before. This time you may like to 'palm the eyes', placing your hands lightly over your closed eyes for a while, then opening your eyes beneath your hands, slowly letting the light filter in as you gradually take the hands away.

If we've been practising concentration as a group we often discuss what we've experienced. Everyone's may be slightly different. There's no 'right' colour, size, etc. Occasionally it just doesn't work for some students, because of the light in the room or some quirk of eyesight. However, people of all ages seem to enjoy candle gazing and we often use it as Christmas approaches.

THE BREATH AS A CONCENTRATION EXERCISE

All breathing exercises are also an exercise in concentration, but this one really focuses the mind. It was a life (or rather, sanity) saver for me during a flight home from a holiday abroad, bringing food poisoning along as unwanted baggage. Counting the breaths stopped me thinking about that sick feeling and the panicky 'what ifs' – 'What if the toilet's occupied?' 'What if the children get it?'

This method involves counting each breath – not the length of the breath, but the breath itself.

Breathe at a normal, quiet rate using the breath of relaxation. Don't make the breathing forced or extra deep. So, a nice easy breath in and out (through the nose) is 1; in and out – 2; in and out – 3; in and out – 4; and then it's back to 1 again.

Very simple, but the mind will want to wander, so you must gently bring it back to the counting. And if it develops the crafty knack of wandering off onto other subjects, and yet you're *still* counting correctly, be more demanding. Picture each number; colour every one differently; draw them in different scripts, and so on – making up ways of resisting that mind which is so adept at running away with us, like a runaway horse.

FURTHER PRACTICE

As this last concentration exercise has shown, the focus of our attention doesn't have to be an immediate physical object. You can let your mind rest on a sound or a word ('peace', 'love' are both popular themes). Or it could be an inspiring piece of music or poetry, a view, a picture, or even a person. Your choice can be as wide as you like and completely personal. Many people who practise concentration/meditation have found that it can add new depth to life.

Nor does concentration practice have to be limited to a set time or place. It can be put into use as you go about your daily life – try to focus on the task in hand and simply *be here now*.

It can transform everyday things. When you're washing up, feel the warmth, the movement of the water, the texture of the crockery, observe the bubbles, the swishing sounds – and so on.

Occasionally while eating, instead of doing it with one eye on the paper and an ear on the radio, sit in silence and slowly savour your meal – even if it's only bread and cheese. You will be able to use your sense of taste and smell as well as the other senses.

Conkers

It may sound as if a concentration exercise is a rather stern and serious thing to do, and it's true that it cannot be done without a little self-discipline. However, I have found that these exercises done with elderly friends have been some of the most enjoyable and enlightening experiences. And when we've chatted over our cups of tea afterwards we've had to admit that our minds come up with some pretty funny things.

Last autumn I produced a mound of freshly-fallen conkers. There were some quizzical looks when the bag was passed around towards the end of class. 'What on earth are we going to do now, have conker fights?' But it turned out to be one of the best 'concentrations' ever, especially among those whose sight was poor. Chestnuts are such tactile things, with their rounded surfaces and waxy, polished skins. It was a familiar object and yet one which many of these pensioners hadn't touched since their childhood, or at least since that of their children.

After we had studied the shape, colour, grain and shine, had felt the morning coolness of them and smelt their lingering woody, acid scent, we closed our eyes and imagined our horse-chestnut resting on the soil, putting down roots, sprouting shoots and leaves and eventually growing into a strong, mature tree – like the one that had shed this seed.

Afterwards there were many reminiscences. For a while discussion centred around the best way to produce a champion fighting conker. Boiling or baking them were popular methods – but was this cheating? At the time such ethics didn't come into it, though. Each child had their special and jealously guarded 'recipe'.

There were other, more peaceful, uses too. Four pins pushed into a conker and two more at the top wound with brightly-coloured cotton make attractive furniture for a doll's house. And did you know that if you put conkers in your drawers they keep the moths out? ('No wonder you sit like that' commented one wit.) By the time the laughter had died down Mrs Blake had fetched proof from her room – 20-year-old conkers, still smooth and glossy, though just a little darker, mahogany instead of chestnut.

A student in a conventional yoga class was a bit nonplussed to be presented with a conker. She explained why afterwards. 'When we had to keep thinking about an apple it was easy – apple tart, apple pie, apple crumble, apple dumplings, baked apple, apple meringue ... Then you handed me a conker tonight and I thought – what on earth can I cook with that?'

Down-to-earth Muriel was about the only student who had no

compunction at all about biting into the apple she'd just been meditating on. Most students find that after really getting to know an object through concentration they feel strangely attached and protective towards it. Flowers tend to be put in water and lamented when they fade. Lucy Behenna pressed hers instead. So perhaps a few conkers will last another 20 years.

CHAPTER 17

SLEEP PROBLEMS

Many older people suffer from sleep problems or insomnia, whether it means having trouble getting to sleep or waking up early and not being able to go back to sleep again. There may be a feeling that the quantity or quality of sleep is not satisfying.

SLEEP PATTERNS

As we get older, sleep patterns change; it is quite normal for sleep to become shorter, lighter and more broken, and usual sleep routines are more easily disturbed. If you have a sleep problem it can be helpful to look at your routine and the amount of sleep you are having. Perhaps you should ask yourself if you are expecting too much – if this is the case, you may need to adjust your expectations and habits.

I know of older people who are tucked up in bed by 9pm and then hope to sleep soundly until 7am. Most are disappointed. They may sleep well from 9.30pm until 4am and then lie awake and restless until it's time to get up. In fact they have had the benefit of 6–7 hours' sleep, which is adequate for most of us, but that sleep has been started too early and it is the long hours from dawn onwards that are remembered and leave the feeling of not having slept long enough. If you recognise this scenario you may be able to work out ways to improve things.

LOOKING AT YOUR ROUTINES

You could try a new routine – going to bed later, passing the extra time with some quiet occupation, such as reading or listening to the radio. Give it a week or so to adapt to the new routine. If you can't hang out that bit longer because you are just too tired, then try changing things at the other end of your sleep time. Instead of lying fretting that you can't recapture sleep, do something positive to fill that time. It might help to actually get up from your bed and take yourself off to another room. Make yourself a drink, read, write letters, listen to a tape – whatever appeals.

Look at the pattern of your day too, as that will affect your sleep. Some things are obvious: are you getting enough fresh air and exercise? could you include more activities which stretch the body and mind so you feel a healthy tiredness at the end of each day? do you doze too much during the day, thus affecting the nightime sleep? (On the other hand, a regular, short daily nap can be helpful, as it may mean that you're not overtired by the end of the day and may be able to go to bed that little bit later, so that your deepest and most beneficial sleep comes at a later, more appropriate time.)

If you have a sleep problem:

- ▶ It is very important to keep regular habits.
- ▶ Avoid excessive daytime napping or long lie-ins in the morning.
- ▶ Try to keep at least *fairly* active during the day.
- ▶ Allow time to 'wind down' in the evening.

THE QUALITY OF YOUR SLEEP

If the *quality* of sleep is unsatisfying you could do more detective work to find the cause. As sleep is more easily disturbed in later life, it is best to avoid those things that can prevent or disrupt sleep, even if they've never been a problem in the past.

- ▶ Are your bed and bedroom comfortable enough?
- ▶ Drink less tea and coffee, especially close to bedtime (more about this later).
- ▶ If you have to get up to go to the toilet during the night, perhaps you should avoid a late night drink. (Frequent visits to the toilet through the night may well be due to a medical problem, especially enlargement of the prostate gland in men, and should be discussed with your doctor.)
- ▶ Avoid the use of alcohol as a sleep-inducer; it can disturb sleep in the latter part of the night.

▶ Is it a medical complaint that hinders sleep? If, for example, you are disturbed by pain, indigestion or breathlessness, see your doctor and explain the problem. Appropriate treatment may mean that you don't have to rely on sleeping pills to make you sleep.

SLEEPING TABLETS

Doctors say it is better to avoid sleeping tablets as they alter the natural cycles of sleep. Sometimes they can be helpful in the short-term, but if you are taking such drugs and want to come off them, don't do it suddenly; see your doctor about cutting down gradually.

GP Angela Gurner says 'Use of hypnotics (sleeping tablets) should be a last resort and a short-term treatment plan of 7–14 days agreed upon before treatment. These drugs have potentially serious side-effects in the elderly, especially confusion and unsteadiness. Not only are we less able to process these drugs effectively as we get older, but sensitivity to their effect is greater and a smaller dose may be required. They carry a greater risk of psychological dependence also.'

LESS WELL KNOWN CAUSES OF SLEEPLESSNESS

There are other, less well known causes of insomnia.

▶ Some prescribed medicines can produce sleeplessness and nightmares.
▶ Diuretics (water tablets) can remain active at night and can also cause night-time cramps. Dosing time may need adjustment.

Discuss these possibilities with your doctor, if you think they may have a bearing on your sleep problems.

PRACTICAL ADVICE FROM A CONSULTANT PSYCHOLOGIST

Dr Marilyn Glenville, a consultant psychologist, outlined her approach to insomnia in our local *Evening Argus*. It is very practical, with a definite yoga flavour and many of my students, of all ages, have benefited from it. Here is the gist of the article, reproduced with Dr Glenville's kind permission:

> Because our mental and physical states are so intertwined, they feed off each other, positively and negatively. If something is worrying us, our bodies become tense and unable to relax. This makes sleep more difficult, which in turn makes us even more stressful. If something physical is stopping us from sleeping, this in turn makes us worried and agitated and then the body becomes more and more tense and tight.

Dr Glenville recommends:

- ▶ Avoiding drinks containing caffeine (tea, coffee, cola) for at least *6 hours* before bed.
- ▶ Avoiding eating for 3 hours.
- ▶ Camomile tea, without milk or sugar, but perhaps with a spoonful of honey, as a bedtime drink.
- ▶ A warm bath or just a warm footbath to relax the body.
- ▶ Soothing music and reading in bed.
- ▶ Tensing every part of the body in turn and then relaxing it (see Systematic Tension Release in Chapter 14, Relaxation).
- ▶ Trying to go to bed in a relaxed frame of mind, leaving daily worries behind.

Blackboard Technique

Dr Glenville suggests trying her *blackboard technique* for when you find getting off to sleep particularly difficult.

- ▶ Lying in bed with your eyes closed, imagine a blackboard. In your imagination see yourself with a piece of chalk in one hand and an eraser in the other.
- ▶ Draw a large circle. Inside the circle put the number 100.

- Use the eraser to rub out the number but be careful not to rub out the circle.
- When you have done that, write the number 99, rub it out as before and continue indefinitely.
- Even if you realise that you've gone back to thinking again, just stop and start from the last number you can remember.

The mind becomes bored with this routine and eventually shuts down. When this is practised over a number of nights, sleep onset becomes quicker and quicker because the mind becomes bored with the routine sooner.

For waking up early, follow the same advice about eating and drinks containing caffeine. Once awake, do the blackboard technique or get out of bed, go to the toilet and then come back to bed and do the technique.

Over the years, I have passed on Dr Glenville's advice to students in yoga and relaxation/meditation classes. Some don't fancy picturing a blackboard, due to schoolday associations, so they adapt it to suit themselves. One student preferred to see the numbers from an overhead projector, another wrote the numbers in the sand, and then watched waves washing them away. Whatever variation is used, quite a number of students have reported back that this technique has worked for them. Lesley was delighted that after a few weeks she only had to think of doing this mental exercise and she was 'out like a light'.

More tips
I would also recommend trying the following:

- Some gentle stretches as described in this book.
- A walk – but not immediately before bed (too stimulating).
- A few drops of relaxing aromatherapy oil – lavender essential oil is a favourite – in the bath or footbath.
- Or dilute the essential oil in a vegetable oil such as almond or grape-seed, and massage into your feet or aching muscles in your neck and shoulders.
- Having let go all over, use the Breath of Relaxation (page 114).
- Try 3 Bee Breaths (page 117).
- Or use The Breath as a Concentration Exercise (page 127).

▶ Look at the herbal and homoeopathic remedies in your chemist – they're non-addictive.
▶ If you have nightmares, try Bach Flower Rescue Remedy, from chemists or health food stores.

All the suggestions given in this chapter have been tried and tested by my students, and feedback has been very encouraging. The list of suggestions to check out is rather long, but out of it you should be able to find a few ideas that will help you if you do suffer from sleep problems.

SUGGESTED PROGRAMMES

All the following programmes last for about 30 to 40 minutes. Each posture, movement or sequence can be repeated as many times as you wish, although three times is the most common choice. Do remember to rest whenever necessary and to work both sides of the body equally.

The programmes are in a progressive order. For example, chest expansion and shoulder exercises in the first few routines pave the way for the more difficult 'cow head' posture in programme 5. However, as we are all different, you may sometimes find a movement in an early programme harder than one in a later programme. Just see how you go.

Move slowly and smoothly. If you feel strain or pain, *stop*. Adapt a posture if necessary, in order to make it more comfortable. Relax and get your breath back between postures.

And remember the golden rule – effort, but not strain.

BASIC PROGRAMME 1

Relaxation
Check your posture – your back should be straight but relaxed. Rest your feet on a cushion if your legs are short. Feel your breath quietening down.

▶ **Action breaths**   Practise deep, smooth breathing, fingertips on shoulders, lifting your elbows as you breathe in and lowering them as you breathe out. Three or six times.

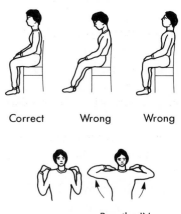

Breathe IN

▶ **Warm up**   Shake and flick hands, then arms, then legs, then wriggle all over.

▶ **Face**   First frown, then relax the brows; lift the brows, then relax them again; purse the lips, then smile.

▶ **Head and neck**   Start with a straight neck, then bend the head forward, chin towards chest. Pause and allow the neck to lengthen, straighten the neck again. Put the head on one side, pause, slowly straighten up again and then repeat to the other side. Look over the shoulder, first to the right, pause, face forwards again, then to the left, as far as the head will comfortably go.

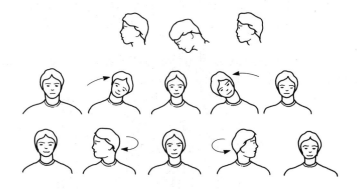

▶ **Swimming**   This is a breast-stroke action in reverse. Breathe in time with the movements. Repeat in reverse order.

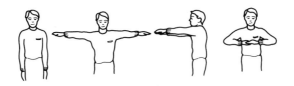

Breathe OUT   Breathe IN   Breathe OUT Breathe IN

▶ **Shoulders** Keeping your arms down, rotate alternate shoulders, lifting and dropping them. Feel the movement with the opposite hand if this helps.
▶ **Hands** Rub your hands together, then clench and stretch out the fingers. Gently pull each finger in turn. Relax the hands, then shake them.

The next two are standing movements

▶ **Leg lift** Check your posture, then lift and lower each leg in turn, first forwards, then to the side, then to the back, keeping the legs straight. Hold onto a chair for support. If you do this sitting down, just lift forwards.

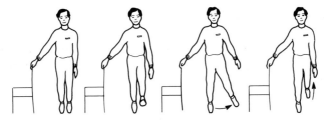

▶ **Side bends** Bend to each side from the waist as far as you can go without bending forward, then straighten up again.

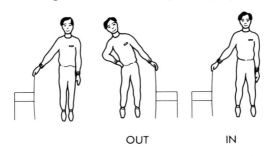

OUT   IN

Now a couple of seated exercises

▶ **Feet**   Rotate your ankles and feet, first one way, then the other.

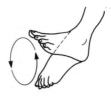

▶ **Relaxation**   Sit comfortably, then methodically tense and relax each part of the body in turn. Allow your thoughts to flow.

PROGRAMME 2

▶ **Relaxation**   Feel the easy flow of the breath of relaxation.

 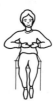

▶ **Breathing awareness**   Place your hands just above the waist. Take long controlled breaths, feeling the body expand as you breathe in, then flattening the tummy and feeling the body becoming smaller and shoulders coming down as you breathe out.
▶ **Action breaths**   Continue the breathing awareness from the previous exercise.

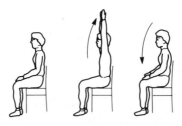

Breathe IN   Breathe OUT

▶ **Warm-up rub**
▶ **Forward bend**
▶ **Backward stretch**

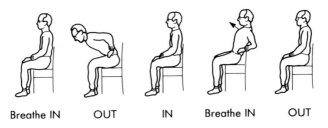

Breathe IN   OUT   IN   Breathe IN   OUT

▶ **Swimming**   Do the breast-stroke action from the basic programme.
▶ **Neck and shoulders**   Again, do the same movements as in the basic programme.
▶ **Leg circling**   Check your standing posture, then circle each leg from the hip. This can also be done from a sitting position.

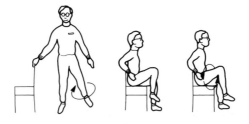

▶ **Squats**   Hold onto a chair back, and slowly squat down on your heels. Then stand up slowly again. If you are seated, do the heel and toe movement.

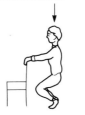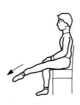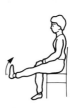

Point toe   Push into heel

▶ **Hands**   Pull and wriggle each finger, then do the finger flop.
▶ **Relaxation**   Feel each part of the body, from the feet upwards, growing heavy and relaxed.

PROGRAMME 3

▶ **Relaxation**   Feel still and quiet at your centre. There should be no feeling of guilt – this is your health investment.

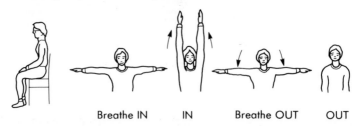

Breathe IN   IN   Breathe OUT   OUT

▶ **Mountain breaths**   Work with your own breathing rate. Do this three or four times.

▶ **Limber up**   Shake each limb, wriggle, etc.

Now some standing movements

▶ **Four-way stretch**   Do this two or three times. Or you could do the seated variation.

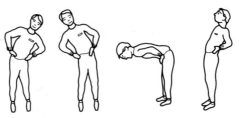

▶ **Squats**   If you are seated, do the knees-up movement.

And now some seated exercises

▶ **Shoulders**   Do some rowing movements, lifting and dropping the shoulders afterwards.

▶ **Neck**   The pendulum movement.

Chin towards chest   Circle chin across chest to look over right shoulder   Make big semi-circle across chest to look over left shoulder

► **Legs** Knee pressing.

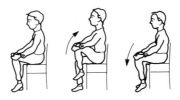

Breathe IN Breathe OUT Breathe IN

► **Hands** Rub and shake them, then pretend you're piano playing. Press the fingers back.
► **Feet** Circle the ankles.
► **Relaxation** Feel each limb becoming warm and heavy. Picture light and warmth spreading out from a centre at your heart.

PROGRAMME 4

► **Relaxation** Feel your friend the breath flowing easily in and out.
► **Action Breaths**

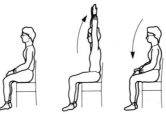

Breathe IN Breathe OUT

► **Limbering up** Flick the hands and feet, shake the limbs.
► **Swimming** Here is a variation on the movement. Lift your arms up to shoulder height in front of you, slowly swing them round behind you, then, clasping your fingers if you can, lift your arms behind you as far as you can without straining. Then lean forward, keeping your arms behind you. Slowly sit up, and relax your arms in front of you.

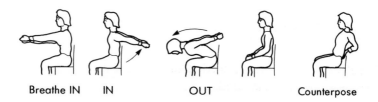

Breathe IN   IN   OUT   Counterpose

▶ **Swimming counterpose**   Rest your hands in the small of your back and lean back. **Or** you could substitute the swimming movement on page 57. This is similar to the variation just described, but starts with the hands in the 'prayer' position and has subtle movement and breathing differences. Counterpose it with a backwards stretch.

▶ **Shoulders**   Circle them forwards three times, then backwards three times, then lift and drop them three times.

Now the standing exercises

▶ **Balance**   Try the tree balance or the stork. If you remain sitting, try knee-pressing.

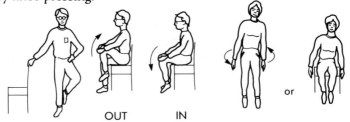

OUT   IN   or

▶ **Hula hoop**   Rotate the hips, pretending you are swinging a hula hoop round. A sitting variation is also possible.

And now the sitting exercises

▶ **Hands**   Pull and stretch your fingers, then shake your hands.

▶ **Feet**   Similarly, pull and stretch your toes, then separate them, and then shake your feet.

▶ **Eyes**   Do the clock movements with your eyes, looking at the various numbers on an imaginary clock-face.

▶ **Breathing**   The bee breath.

▶ **Relaxation**   Let go from the forehead down, finishing with your toes.

▶ **Visualisation**   Visualise your favourite place.

PROGRAMME 5

A belt or a scarf might be needed for some of these exercises. And have some music to hand.

▶ **Relaxation**   Rest your hands on your tummy, and feel the gentle rise and fall during the breath of relaxation.
▶ **Controlled breathing awareness**   Now feel the stronger lift of your tummy when you breathe in and the greater fall as you consciously flatten your tummy as you breathe out.

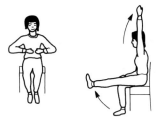

▶ **Stretches**   As in the basic programme 1.
▶ **Hornpipe**   Place one arm across the front of your waist and the other across the back, then reverse the movement. Keep repeating this smoothly.

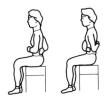

▶ **Cow head**   You can use a scarf or a belt for this one if your hands don't reach each other behind your back.

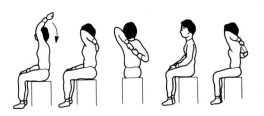

▶ **Shoulders**   Loosen them off by circling them forwards three times, then backwards three times, then lift and drop them three times.

▶ **Neck**   Do the chicken neck, then lower your head from side to side; then look over each shoulder.

Now a standing exercise

▶ **Four-way stretch**   Or you can do the seated variation.

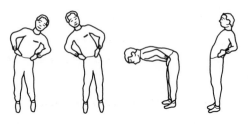

And now sitting

▶ **Legs and hips**   Circle the legs from the hips.
▶ **Breathing**   The tension-releasing breath.
▶ **Relaxation**   Let go throughout the body, from top to toe.
▶ **Visualisation**   Play some music and see yourself moving easily or dancing to it.

PROGRAMME 6

▶ **Relaxation**   Sit and just feel everything slowing down and becoming quiet.

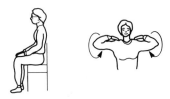

▶ **Elbows**   With your hands on your shoulders, circle your elbows in time with your breathing.

▶ **Swimming in space**   Bring your palms together in front of you, raise them together to the ceiling as you breathe in, then sweep them down by your sides as you breathe out.

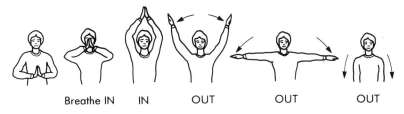

Breathe IN   IN   OUT   OUT   OUT

▶ **Tarzan impression**   Breathe in, then while you're breathing out thump your chest and let out an echoing Tarzan cry. Don't feel inhibited.

Now a couple of movements for your shoulders

▶ With your hands behind your neck, bring your elbows together in front of you.

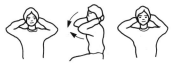

▶ **Rowing**   With your arms out in front of you, make fists of your hands, as if you were holding oars. Then as you breathe out, bend your elbows and bring your fists towards your chest. Reverse the movement, breathing in.

Two more movements for your neck

▶ Drop your chin forwards and down and rest it there. Then lift it back up. Then drop your head slowly to one side then to the other.
▶ **Owl visualisation**   See page 110.

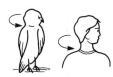

▶ **Hands**   Press each finger (between joints) towards your palm, then press them away from you.

▶ **Wrists** Move your hands round in a circle, first one way, then the other.

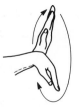

▶ **The cat** This can either be done in the standing position, holding on to the back of a chair, or you can do it sitting down. Or you can even try it in the original position, on the floor.

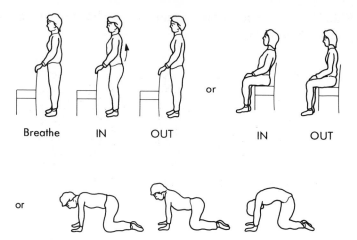

Breathe   IN   OUT   or   IN   OUT

or   Breathe IN   Breathe OUT

▶ **Sitting** Try exercising some of those odd places, for example by tummy tightening or by trying the pelvic-floor exercises.
▶ **Feet** Circle the ankles both together, first one way, then the other, and then shake your feet well.
▶ **Relaxation** Let go from the toes upwards.
▶ **Visualisation** See your troubles being placed, one by one, in a hot-air balloon, which then floats away.

PROGRAMME 7

▶ **Relaxation**   Calm your thoughts by focusing on your breath. 'Watch' it coming and going, but don't try to deepen it or control it.

▶ **Warm up**   Try a warm-up thump and perhaps the Tarzan cry from the previous programme.

▶ Do some good stretches, and/or **swimming in space**.

Now the standing movements

▶ Try a **cat variation**   If you find it too much standing, do it in the sitting position.

▶ **Side bends** or **half moon**   Again, this can be done in the seated position if necessary.

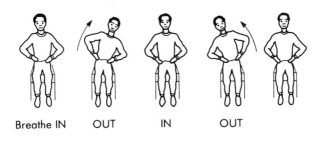

Breathe IN   OUT   IN   OUT

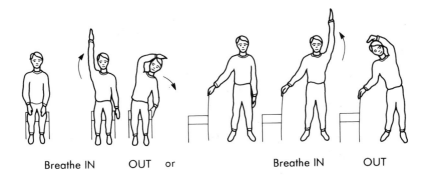

Breathe IN   OUT   or   Breathe IN   OUT

Sitting movements

▶ **Neck**   Roll your head like a pendulum across your chest.
▶ **Shoulders**   Pretend you are stirring the pud, polishing the table or cleaning windows. Finish off by lifting and dropping your shoulders a few times.
▶ **Sitting twist**   Cross one leg over the other and twist round and look over your shoulder. And don't forget to repeat the movement on the other side.

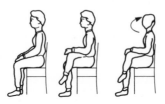

▶ **Rag doll**   Flop forwards and completely relax, breathing out with a 'Ha' as you go forwards.

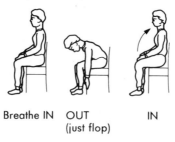

Breathe IN   OUT   IN
              (just flop)

▶ **Relaxation**   Let yourself go from top to toe.
▶ **Visualisation**   Picture yourself walking in the countryside.

PROGRAMME 8

You may need an extra chair for this programme.

▶ **Relaxation**   Tune in to how you are feeling today. Let any negative feelings flow out with the breath. Breathe the opposite, positive, feeling in. For example, breathe out tiredness, breathe in energy.
▶ **Mountain breaths**   Do three or six of these.

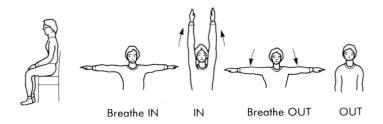

Breathe IN   IN   Breathe OUT   OUT

▶ **Limbering up** Try some flicks, some knees-up, some floor stomps, etc.

▶ **Neck** Drop your chin forward, rest there, then lift your head up. Now drop your head from side to side. Look over each shoulder.

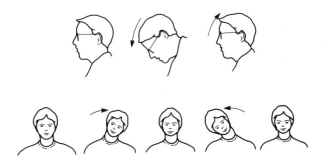

▶ **Arms** Do some elbow snaps.

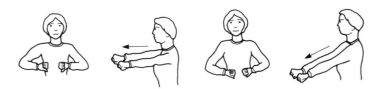

▶ **Shoulders** Lift and drop your shoulders a few times.

Here are some exercises that can be done sitting on two chairs or on the floor

▶ **Stretches** Towards the toes, remembering to breathe out as you lean forward and let the knees bend a little as necessary.

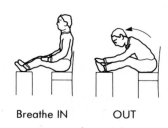

Breathe IN   OUT

▶ **Forward bends**   You can do these either with your hands sliding along your legs or with your arms raised above your head. Use a cushion under your tail if seated on the floor.

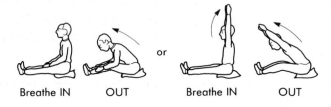

Breathe IN   OUT   *or*   Breathe IN   OUT

▶ **Backwards stretch**   This counterbalances the forward bends.

Breathe IN

▶ **Knee bends**   Bend the right knee and straighten it three times, then repeat three times with the left knee.

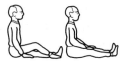

Breathe OUT Breathe IN

▶ **Breathing**   Sitting normally, allow the breath to settle. Feel the out breaths growing a little longer than the in breaths.
▶ **Relaxation**   Count down your breaths from ten to one to reach a deeper level of relaxation.
▶ **Visualisation**   Picture any soothing scene and see yourself well and happy. Count your breaths back from one to ten to bring yourself round.

QUESTIONS PEOPLE ASK

Q *I wear a spinal corset. What exercises can I do?*

A Gentle stretches are good. Leave out any twisting movements and ones that round the back – rag doll for example. However it would probably not be advisable to exercise without the support of your corset.

Q *I can't fit the breathing in at the same time as doing a sequence of movements.*

A Sometimes it helps to make these movements a little faster to fit in with your breathing rate. If this doesn't work, concentrate for the time being on only doing the movements and let your breath 'do its own thing'. Be sure, though, that you do *keep breathing* – lots of people hold their breath while concentrating hard.

Q *One of my arms won't lift very far. How can I encourage it?*

A Use the good arm to help the other. Rest the hand of the weaker arm on that of the stronger. Lift both arms as far as the weaker one will go without causing strain or pain. Or hold a stick between the hands and use it in the same way. Or a *sensitive* helper can slowly lift it for you, but let them know just how far to go. (See Chapter 8)

Q *I've got a weak leg.*

A A weaker leg can be helped in the same way, this time by crossing the ankles, stronger leg at the bottom, and using the good leg to lift the weaker one. Or lift it by pulling on the trouser leg. Or you can do the same thing using a wide belt or strap. Or again a helper could raise it carefully for you.

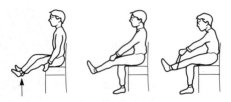

Q *How often should I do the exercises and for how long at a time?*

A This really is up to you – and your fitness, time available and dedication. Most elderly people find the average 30-minute programme described in this book is quite long enough (remember that each programme includes time for relaxation and pauses between exercises). If in doubt start with 10 or 20 minutes at a time and build up. Some elderly students just do a full session once or twice a week. Others do 10 or 20 minutes daily. Some do things when they think of them during the day – action breaths and stretches on waking, foot movements while the adverts are on TV, neck, shoulder and hand movements after time spent sewing, relaxation and visualisation in bed at night to help get to sleep.

Q *Don't you think it's best to have a rigid timetable to make sure we do our exercises every day?*

A It is good to set aside a regular time and place, but try to remain flexible. Sometimes allow for illness, busy or 'off' days, otherwise such failures may put you off completely.

Q *How can I tell if I'm overdoing it?*

A Such exercise shouldn't cause pain. If it does, then you're overdoing it. Also, if you feel breathless during the session or end it with a flat feeling of exhaustion instead of a sense of well-being you will know that it has been too strenuous or lengthy for you.

Q *My hip (or knee) hurts when I practise some of the standing exercises. What should I do?*

A Taking all the weight on one leg while you raise, rotate or balance on the other can be a strain. You would be better advised to do the leg movements from a seated position.

Q *I have arthritis. Is it safe for me to try some of your exercises?*

A Such movements can be very helpful for arthritis sufferers. But play close attention to how your body feels as you do them and stop if there is pain. *Don't* exercise a joint while it is inflamed. (See Chapter 5.)

Q *Help! My neck creaks when I turn it, my shoulders crackle when I move them and my knee-bends sound like gunfire!*

A Rest assured. You are not alone! We all crackle and creak a bit – some more than others. Unless it is accompanied by pain, just don't worry about it.

Q *I go dizzy when I get up from the chair/floor/bed. Why is this?*

A We all have this sensation if we jump up too quickly, and some people are more prone to it than others. It's all to do with our blood pressure having to adjust as we move from one position to another. Older people are affected more and have to take plenty of time over such movements, doing it by degrees and pausing when necessary. (See Chapter 5). Use the method shown on page 97 when getting up from the floor.

Q *I can still touch my toes if I do it quickly. Why won't you let me?*

A See the question and answer above – that's one reason. Another is that you could hurt yourself before you realise it with such a quick and jerky movement – your back is especially vulnerable. And you wouldn't have time to use your spine in the correct, safe way that we teach for a forward bend. Anyway, an important principle of these yoga-type exercises is that it's not how *far* you go that matters, but the *way* that you do it.

Q *I get a bit constipated and am taking a higher fibre diet that my doctor suggested. Will exercise help too?*

A Swimming, dancing will all help a sluggish digestive system. Many of the movements described in this book also give the abdominal organs a gentle squeeze or massage. Forward bends, twists, the cat, and particularly the bellows, will all stimulate this area, as will the more subtle tummy and pelvic-floor exercises. (See Chapter 11.)

Physiotherapists have found that massaging your abdomen helps to 'get things moving'. This is best done lying on your back with knees bent and feet flat on the bed. Have the tummy uncovered and use a massage oil if you like.

Start on the lower right hand side of your abdomen, move your hand up, then across about waist level, then down the left-hand side, finishing here. Lightly sweep your hand across the skin back to the starting point. Repeat several times. Rolling a soft small ball over your tummy in the same way has been found a simple and effective form of abdominal massage.

I suggest you try abdominal exercises then massage as a daily routine. There is no set frequency for the massage and 'as often as you fancy' is the general advice.

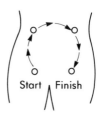

Q *I sometimes get cramp in my legs when I'm exercising, and sometimes during the night. What would you recommend?*

A The best way to relieve the cramped muscle is to stretch it gently. If it is in the back of your calf straighten your leg, pushing into your heel (the opposite of pointing your toes). For night cramps of the calf, get up and walk about for a few minutes. A hot bath before bed can help to prevent them. A rather strange but effective treatment for cramp, *wherever it is occuring in the body*, is to massage firmly the 'pressure point' for cramp, which is between the base (the web) of the big toe and its neighbour. However it is not advisable to do this if you are diabetic or have very fragile skin. Cramps after exercise can be avoided by building up the exercise slowly over several weeks. It is important to warm up before vigorous exercise by doing a few simple stretches and to cool down slowly afterwards. General advice is to take more vitamin E, as this can reduce cramps, as can anything that helps to improve circulation – exercise and massage, for example. Practising relaxation can help too. Some people recommend drinking tonic water (which contains quinine). We have found that the Biochemic Tissue Salt Mag Phos can be a great help if there is a tendency to cramps (from some chemists and health food stores). Diuretics (water tablets) can sometimes cause cramps. If the problem is severe or persists, take advice from your doctor.

Useful Addresses

There are many forms of help available to older people either living alone or with a family:

▶ Supplementary benefits if you are in financial need
▶ Home helps
▶ Home nursing
▶ Aids and appliances
▶ Cheap and special transport
▶ Laundry services
▶ Clubs and holiday schemes

Departments of Social Services, Age Concern groups, old people's welfare committees and Citizens' Advice Bureaux can all give information about these and other kinds of help. You will find addresses in the telephone directory.

Help the Aged

Help the Aged is a national organisation set up to promote the well-being of older people. If you contact them they will be able to offer a wide range of advice and information.

Help the Aged, 1 St James Walk, London EC1R OBE. Tel: 071-253 0253 or call **Senior Line**, they 'Know everything to do with retirement'. Freephone no: 0800 289 404 Mon.–Fri. 10am–4pm.

Age Concern

Age Concern England is a similar organisation to Help the Aged, except that there are also local groups operating throughout the country. You can find the address of your nearest Age Concern group in the telephone directory, or contact their head office at:

Age Concern England, Astral House, 1268 London Road, London SW16 4ER. Tel: 081-679 8000

Centre for Policy on Ageing

This is an independent unit set up to promote better services for older people. An integral part of the CPA's work is the provision of information to those who work with older people, and its library and information service is widely used. A useful publication of theirs is *Staying Active*.

Centre for Policy on Ageing, 25–31 Ironmonger Row, London EC1V 3QP Tel: 071–253 1787

The Sports Council

They have a leaflet, *50+ All to Play For*, giving general advice on exercise. They also can give you the address of the governing body of any specific sport you may be interested in. The Sports Council also have regional offices.

The Sports Council, 16 Upper Woburn Place, London WC1H OQP Tel: 071–388 1277

EXTEND – Exercise Training for the Elderly and Disabled.

Extend was set up to provide a specially graded series of exercises for the elderly and disabled, promoting health and fitness through recreational movement. The exercise classes are actually set up under the umbrella of local organisations such as the health and social services, over 60s' clubs, day centres, and are linked together by newsheets, letters, etc.

EXTEND Exercise Training Limited, 22 Maltings Drive, Wheathampstead, Herts. AL4 8QJ Tel: 0582 832760

The Beth Johnson Foundation

This organisation will provide ideas for activities that can be taken up after retirement. It also has a useful range of publications.

The Beth Johnson Foundation, Parkfield House, 64 Princes Road, Hartshill, Stoke on Trent, ST4 7JL Tel: 0782 44036

The British Wheel of Yoga
The aims of the Wheel are:

▶ to encourage and help all persons to a greater knowledge and understanding of yoga and its practice through the provision of study, education and training;
▶ to maintain and improve the standard of teaching;
▶ to cooperate with and support other organisations which have similar aims. Activities include public meetings, seminars, the supervision of yoga teacher training, cooperation with local education authorities in the provision of yoga classes, and the publication of a wide range of literature. As well as 57 County Representatives, who supervise work in their respective counties, there is a Central Office.

The British Wheel of Yoga, 1 Hamilton Place, Boston Road, Sleaford, Lincs NG34 7ES Tel: 0529 306851

Yoga for Health Foundation
The Yoga for Health Foundation is a somewhat smaller organisation than the Wheel of Yoga, but it does specialise in remedial yoga – yoga designed to help those with specific physical problems. They are noted for helping sufferers of multiple sclerosis.

Yoga for Health Foundation, Ickwell Bury, Biggleswade, Beds. SG18 9EF Tel: 0767 627271

The Yoga Biomedical Trust
The YBT operates under the guidance and auspices of professionals of international standing. Its doctors, yoga therapists and researchers are dedicated to the study of yoga as a therapy in the treatment and prevention of specific diseases and conditions, including asthma and diabetes, heart conditions, high blood pressure, stroke and brain damage, Parkinson's disease, low back pain, stress/life crisis intervention. There is a yoga therapy clinic in London.

Yoga Biomedical Trust, PO Box 140, Cambridge CB4 3SY Tel: 0223 67301

Yoga Therapy Clinic, Royal London Homoeopathic Hospital, 60 Great Ormond St, London WC1N 3HR Tel: 071–833 7267

Listening for Health

Matthew Manning, the well known healer, produces a series of Listening for Health audio cassettes which provide information about various problems and which use relaxation and visualisation as aids to self-healing. Titles include:

- ▶ Relieving Osteoarthritis
- ▶ Resisting Allergies
- ▶ Relief from Insomnia
- ▶ Laugh Your Way to Health
- ▶ Just Relax

New Age Innovations, PO Box 602, Ilford, Essex, 1G3 8EP Tel: 081–597 9999

The Cancer Help Centre

This is the well publicised Bristol Cancer Help Centre that provides a wide range of therapies and assistance to cancer sufferers of all ages.

Cancer Help Centre, Cornwallis Grove, Clifton, Bristol BS8 4PG Tel: 0272 743216

Disabled Living Foundation

The foundation has a centre for aids and a very useful information service available to the disabled.

Disabled Living Foundation, 380–384 Harrow Road, London W9 2HU. Tel: 071–289 6111

The Pain Relief Foundation

The Pain Relief Foundation's Pain Research Institute produce an excellent audio cassette called *Coping with Pain*. It is presented by Magnus Magnussun with an introduction by Simon Weston. Side one is called *How to Cope with Pain* and side two is entitled *Relaxation for Pain Relief*. Price £7.55 (including P&P). They also produce audio cassettes on *Coping with Back Pain* and *Coping with Headaches and Migraine*. The book *In Pain? A self-help guide for chronic pain sufferers* by Dr Chris Wells and Graham Nown, Optima Books, £7.99 + £1.50 p+p, is also available from them. Their address is WLAP, PO Box 1, Wirral, L47 7DD.

Self Help and Support Groups

Whatever health problem you, your relative or friend is suffering from, there is probably an organisation to help. The groups cover conditions such as: arthritis, asthma, cancer, diabetes, heart disease, stroke, Parkinson's disease, tinnitus, tranquilliser problems, mental disorders, nervous problems and partial sightedness or hardness of hearing.

The relevant organisation or self help group can provide you with information, practical advice, support and social opportunities. Your local library will have a comprehensive list of both national and local organisations (you can visit or telephone). Your doctor's surgery and the local telephone (Thompson) directory will also include some details.

INDEX

ABOUT THE AUTHOR

MARGARET GRAHAM has lived and worked among a lively elderly community for over thirty years. Her parents founded a charitable home – Ifield Park – pioneering an environment which encouraged an active and independent old age.

Her interest and involvement in yoga began after her doctor prescribed yoga to alleviate a back problem. She developed a programme of modified yoga movements to share the enjoyment and benefit with her older friends.

These highly successful classes are still thriving many years later at a number of homes and care centres.

Margaret Graham, a qualified British Wheel of Yoga teacher, is in great demand for lectures, demonstrations and training sessions in her method as well as instructing conventional yoga classes for adult education centres. She has also written a number of magazine articles on the benefits of yoga for old and young.

A keen cyclist and lifelong vegetarian, she lives in Sussex with her husband, two grown-up daughters and young son.